Oklahoma Health Center
A History

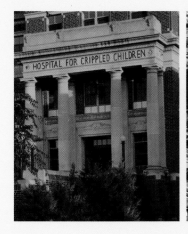
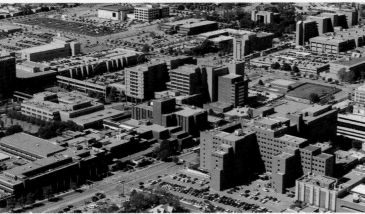
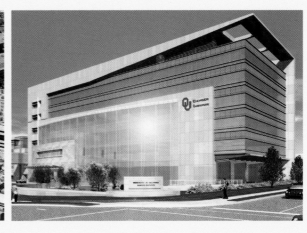

Oklahoma Health Center–A History

By Bob Burke

SERIES EDITOR
Gini Moore Campbell
ASSOCIATE EDITORS
Eric Dabney & Christopher A. Gordon

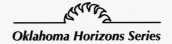

Oklahoma Horizons Series

Printed in the United States of America by Baker Group, LLC-405.503.3207

ISBN: 1-885596-76-6
         978-1-885596-76-5
Library of Congress Control Number: 2009923168
Designed by Skip McKinstry

Oklahoma Health Center—A History

Acknowledgments

Telling the story of the institutions that comprise the Oklahoma Health Center was a massive project. Thankfully, Robert Hardy, the author of the early history of OHC, spent years interviewing the major players in the development of the campus and accumulated a huge body of research before his death. This book could not have been written without the help of many people.

Hershel Lamirand, president of the Oklahoma Health Center Foundation, and his exemplary assistant, Mary Kay Audd, guided the project with precision. They made the way easy to interview the CEOs and directors of campus institutions. Cooperation was splendid.

The leaders of the institutions not only proofread the manuscript, but offered assistance of many staff members. We are thankful to Judy Kelley, editor of OU Medicine; Diane Clay and Cheryl Ottman at the OU Health Sciences Center; Lori Webster at the Oklahoma School of

Science and Mathematics; Clinton M. "Marty" Thompson, Jr., and Mark Hopkins at the Robert M. Bird Health Sciences Library; Terri Folks and Terry Taylor at the Oklahoma Health Center Foundation; Chidindu Aderibigbe at the VA Medical Center; Lisa Mallory at the Oklahoma Allergy and Asthma Clinic; and Gayle Lipscomb at the OU College of Medicine.

Linda Lynn, Melissa Hayer, Mary Phillips, Robin Davison, and Billie Harry at the Oklahoma Publishing Company provided photographs. Michael Dean, William Welge, Rodger Harris, and Bill Moore at the Oklahoma Historical Society gave research assistance. Research and writing was guided by Oklahoma Heritage Association series editor Gini Moore Campbell and associate editors Eric Dabney and Christopher A. Gordon.

Bob Burke
2009

Oklahoma Health Center
A History

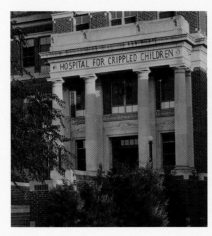
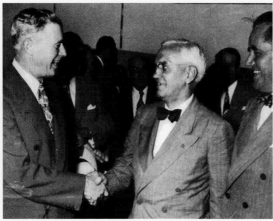
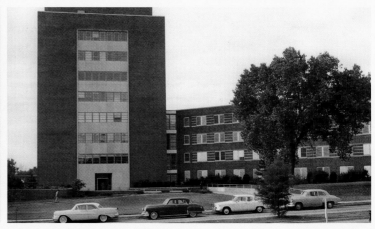

Chapter One

What's In A Name?

The Oklahoma Health Center (OHC) perhaps has made the largest impact upon Oklahoma's economy of any project in the state's first century, including the massive infusion of jobs and federal government spending at Tinker Air Force Base. Yet "Oklahoma Health Center" is not a household name among citizens and business and government leaders. Dr. G. Rainey Williams, a pioneer in the development of the OHC, said many years ago that it was the "best kept secret in Oklahoma." There are good reasons.

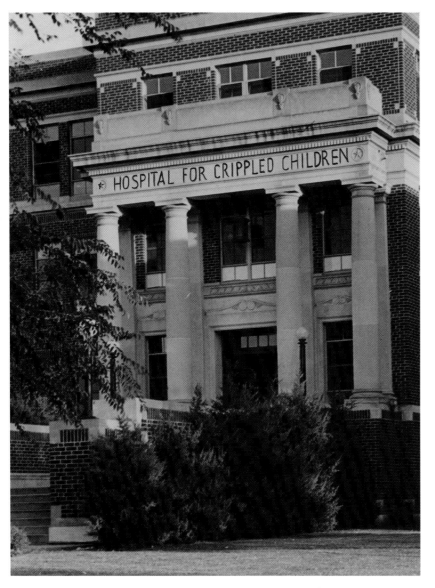

The Crippled Children's Hospital was the major center for treatment of children with severe diseases during the Great Depression. *Courtesy Oklahoma Publishing Company.*

The OHC campus south of the State Capitol has housed health care facilities for nearly a century. The University of Oklahoma (OU) College of Medicine was founded in the area in 1900 and the original University Hospital was built on Northeast 13th Street in 1919. Because OU was the only occupant of the area for decades, the area became known as the "Medical Center" or, simply, the "Med Center."

Even after the Oklahoma Medical Research Foundation and the Veterans Administration Hospital joined University and Children's Hospital and the OU health professional training colleges in the corridor, the area still was referred to as the Med Center. In 1971, university officials formally changed the name of university-related facilities to the OU Health Sciences Center. The new name was often incorrectly used to describe the entire area, not just the university buildings and programs. At present, a prominent sign, "OU Medical Center," at the corner of Northeast 13th Street and Lincoln Boulevard, identifies the hospitals and OUHSC identifies the teaching schools. However, many believe the entire area is still the Med Center.

In the late 1970s, as the area was becoming a multi-institutional health campus, officials spent six months trying to create a more distinctive and descriptive name. Without success, "Oklahoma Health Center" remains the official name of the sprawling 300-acre campus that has literally transformed a blighted Oklahoma City neighborhood into the unique epicenter of health care, education, research, technology, and community services organizations.

OHC represents a $3 billion capital investment. The member institutions provide nearly 13,000 jobs as the state's second-largest employer. Studies show the annual economic impact of OHC is nearly $2 billion. That impact is expected to grow exponentially in the next generation.

The incredible success of OHC can be traced to the cooperation of privately-owned health care providers and research institutions, OU, and government and business leaders. The finest efforts in research, medicine, education, and technology have been pooled to provide cutting-edge health care for Oklahomans and the entire world. The work of practicing and teaching physicians and research scientists helps fuel interactive disciplines within the complex to create an exciting, dynamic environment for health—both now and in the future.

This blend of government, university, and private cooperation did not happen overnight—nor did it come easy. It became a reality because of the work of visionary leaders who saw deep into the hearts of Oklahomans and dreamed of programs and services that many considered to be impossible dreams.

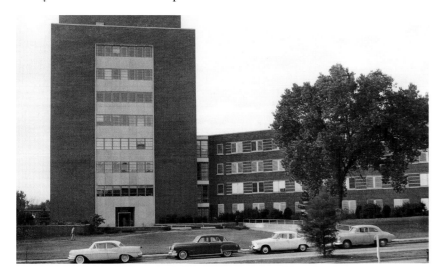

The latest addition to University Hospital in 1959 included laboratory space and patient rooms. *Courtesy Oklahoma Publishing Company.*

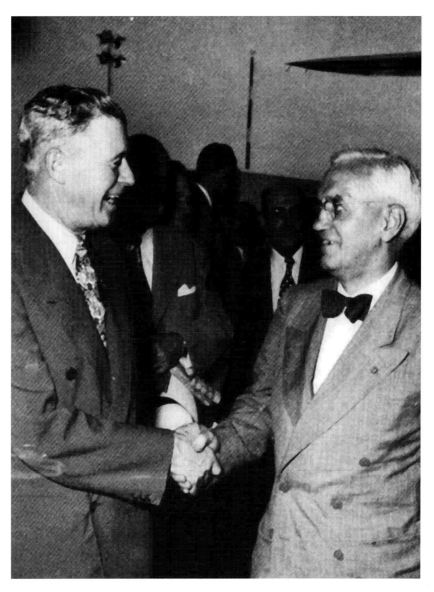

The inventor of penicillin, Sir Alexander Fleming, right, was the guest of honor for the dedication of the Oklahoma Medical Research Foundation, held prior to its completion in 1949. *Courtesy Oklahoma Publishing Company.*

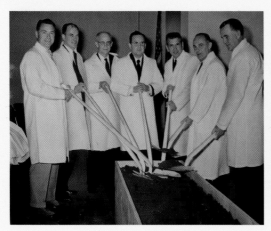 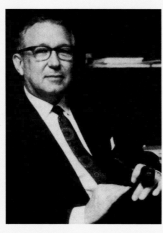 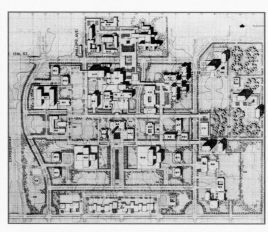 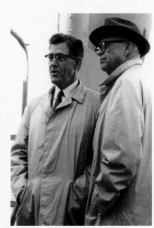

Chapter Two

An Idea Is Born

The idea that became
the Oklahoma Health Center
was birthed in the vision and dreams of five
Oklahoma City civic and medical leaders
who were confronted with a unique set of
problems and circumstances in the 1960s.
The "fathers" of the OHC were Dean A. McGee,
Stanton L. Young, Harvey P. Everest,
E.K. Gaylord, and Dr. Don O'Donoghue.

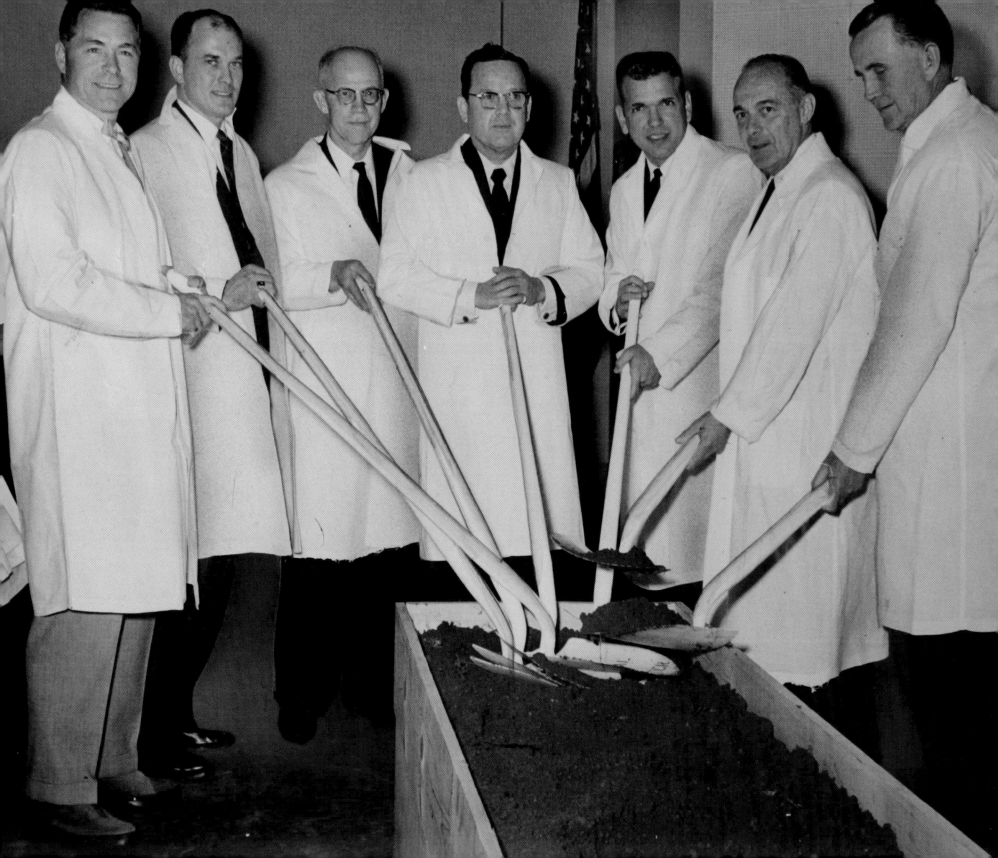

There were rumors that the OU College of Medicine, the only medical school in the state, was at risk to lose its accreditation. Leaders knew that would be a devastating blow to the state's image and the future of training health care workers. There were many reasons the medical school was in financial trouble, but at the heart of the crisis was the lack of state funding to provide adequate educational and research space.

In addition to the threat of losing medical school accreditation, the board of Wesley Hospital also was facing funding difficulties. Doctors at the Oklahoma City Clinic, who had close ties with Wesley Hospital, called for an upgrade and expansion of the facility. The 190-bed hospital at Northwest 12th Street and Harvey Avenue was more than 50 years old, having opened in 1910.

Ironically, many of the trustees of the foundation that governed Wesley Hospital were members of Westminster Presbyterian Church in Oklahoma City, led by Pastor Ray Campbell. Members interested in the future of Wesley Hospital were business and civic leader Stanton L. Young and oilmen Dean A. McGee and John Kirkpatrick.

Often, conversation in Pastor Campbell's office turned to possible solutions to expand Wesley Hospital. The Oklahoma City Clinic nor the hospital had sufficient funds to grow, so the board turned to the state Presbyterian leadership. After a difficult campaign, the Presbyterians approved the idea of taking control of Wesley Hospital, changing the name to Presbyterian Hospital in 1964.

Immediately, Young, the chairman of the Presbyterian Hospital board, and his fellow board members began looking for a new location to build a larger hospital and expand its community role. Baptist Hospital had built a new facility in far northwest Oklahoma City, so Presbyterian leaders looked for land closer to the inner city and its client base.

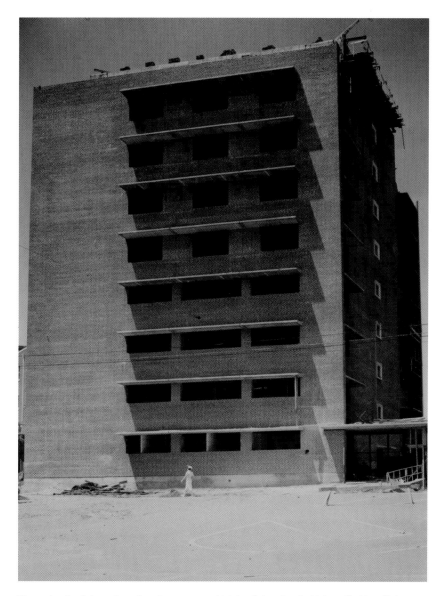

(Left) At a groundbreaking for a new $800,000 research building at the OU Medical Center in 1960 are, left to right, Oklahoma City Mayor James Norick, Representative Bryce Baggett, OU College of Medicine Dean Dr. Mark Everett, OU Regent T.R. Benedum, Lieutenant Governor George Nigh, Dr. Paul Weiss, and OU President Dr. George L. Cross. *Courtesy Oklahoma Publishing Company.*

The outpatient department and neuro-psychiatric clinic wing to University Hospital was completed in 1951. *Courtesy Oklahoma Publishing Company.*

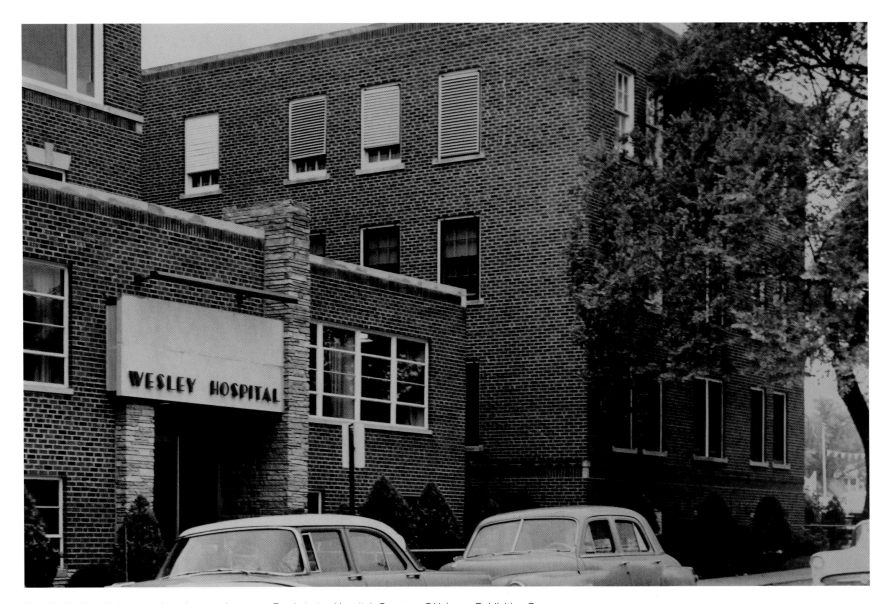

The Wesley Hospital, in 1959, later became known as Presbyterian Hospital. *Courtesy Oklahoma Publishing Company.*

In addition to gaining support for a new, expanded Presbyterian Hospital, the idea of saving the OU College of Medicine rallied business leaders. An important part of the plan was to hire the right person as the new dean of the OU College of Medicine. Dr. James L. "Jim" Dennis, a quiet and gentle pediatrician, became dean of the medical school in 1964. Although he was born and raised in Britton, a north Oklahoma City suburb, and received his medical degree from OU, he had been professor of pediatrics at the University of Arkansas College of Medicine in Little Rock.

Dennis interviewed for the job only a week following gall bladder surgery and still was somewhat shaky when he met with the search committee chaired by Dr. Leonard Eliel, president of the Oklahoma Medical Research Foundation (OMRF). What Dennis found was an underfunded medical center with "good people who did not have adequate facilities." From the beginning, he was impressed with the dedication of doctors, nurses, and other health care professionals.

However, Dennis was disappointed in the condition of University Hospital. He was appalled by the lack of updating and maintenance. In fact, the hospital had deteriorated from Dennis' days as a student at OU a quarter century before. He was overwhelmed by the stench from a single urinal—a hole in the floor with a tin drain that served 27 male patients in one of the wards.

Although Dennis could not brag about what he found, he saw incredible potential. He met with citizens from around the state who were interested in improving health care. It was apparent to him that Oklahomans could receive better health care if more doctors, nurses, dentists, technicians, and other health professionals were trained. At the time, there was a nationwide shortage of 50,000 doctors. Since the beginning of World War II, the demand

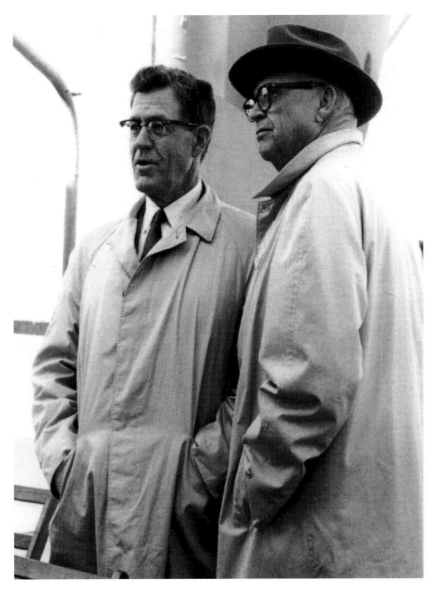

Dean A. McGee, left, and United States Senator Robert S. Kerr had great influence in the federal government and helped early efforts to acquire federal funding for development of the Oklahoma Health Center. *Courtesy Oklahoma Publishing Company.*

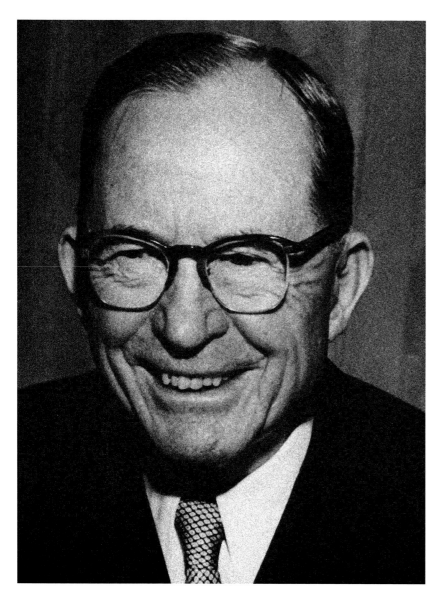

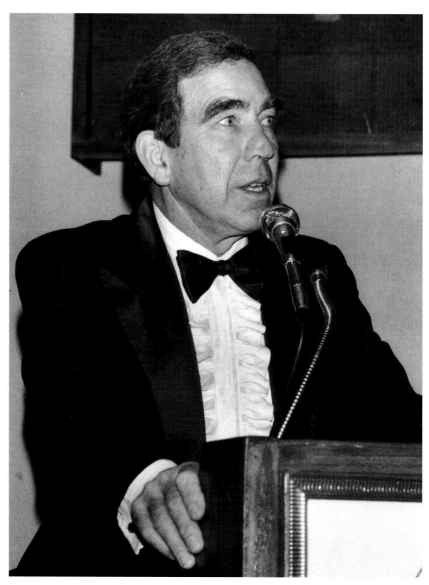

Publisher E.K. Gaylord used the power of the press to influence Oklahomans to support the idea of a comprehensive medical center in Oklahoma City. *Courtesy Oklahoma Publishing Company.*

Dr. William G. "Bill" Thurman was a major player in mapping plans to expand the Oklahoma Health Center campus. *Courtesy Oklahoma Publishing Company.*

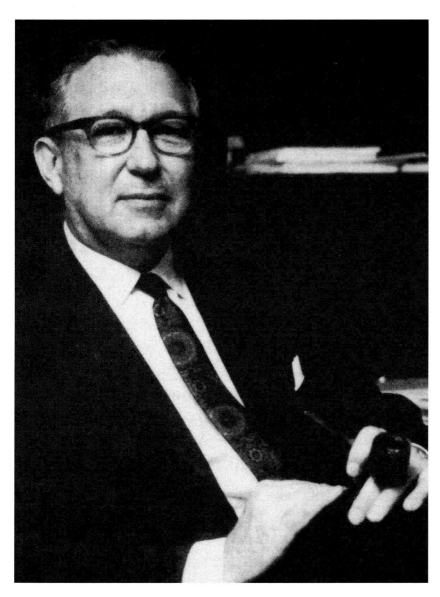

Dr. James L. Dennis came to the OU College of Medicine in 1964 as dean and made a huge difference in the progress of plans for the Oklahoma Health Center. *Courtesy University of Oklahoma.*

for nurses had exceeded the supply. There was serious understaffing in every category of health care in Oklahoma.

Dennis recognized that little legislative attention had been granted the Medical Center during the previous decades. University Hospital opened in 1919 after the legislature decided to forego adding a dome to the State Capitol in favor of building a hospital for the OU College of Medicine. The building that eventually became known as "Old Main" was the result of $219,000 in state appropriations in 1917 and 1919. However, since 1919, little improvement had been made.

There were no private rooms. The simple structure had large wards with beds arranged in non-military fashion. Medical problems discussed with a patient were easily overheard by fellow patients in adjacent beds. Large four-feet square blower fans attempted to cool the hospital, although the moving air made infection control nearly impossible. The hospital survived by using student nurses and crash courses were given to medical students so they could serve as nursing assistants.

The state of the Children's Hospital was not much better. Opened in 1928, equipment was outdated and staffing was woefully short. When Lloyd Rader, director of the Oklahoma Department of Public Welfare, visited Dr. Dennis in the medical school, housed in the yellow brick building built in 1928 on the corner of Northeast 13th Street and Phillips Avenue, he found the medical school budget so tight that Dennis had no money to buy a typewriter. Rader loaned one to Dennis and began to believe in the new voice of the Medical Center.

In Dennis' first few days on the job, he met with federal officials who were reviewing applications for federal matching funds to build a new University Hospital. Almost immediately, Dennis

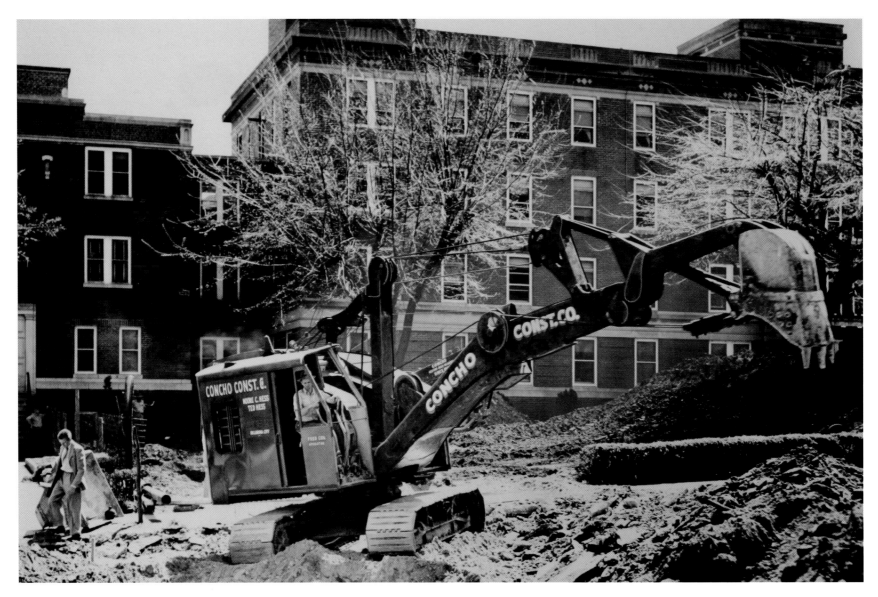

Heavy equipment digs a tunnel in 1950 to connect University Hospital and the new Oklahoma Medical Research Foundation Building. *Courtesy Oklahoma Publishing Company.*

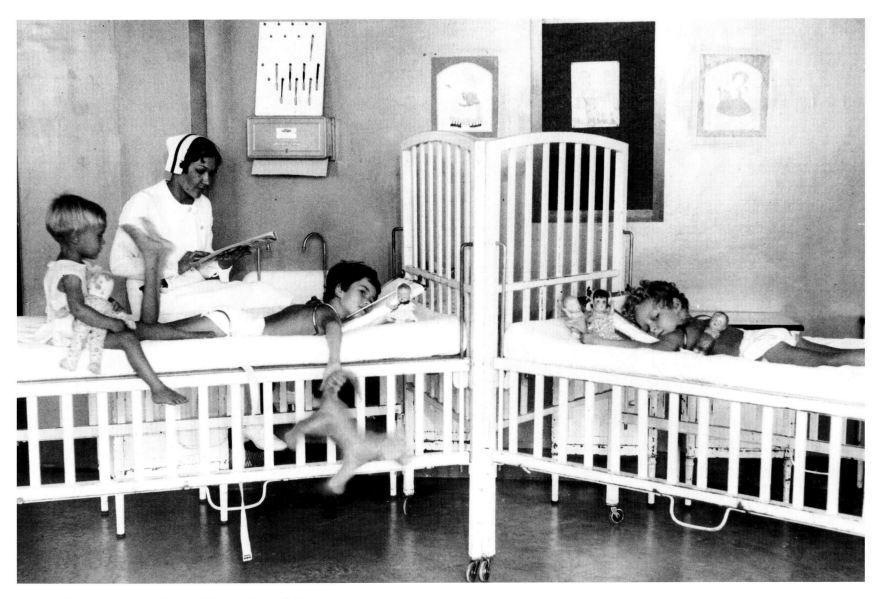

A children's treatment ward at Children's Memorial Hospital in 1933. *Courtesy Oklahoma Publishing Company.*

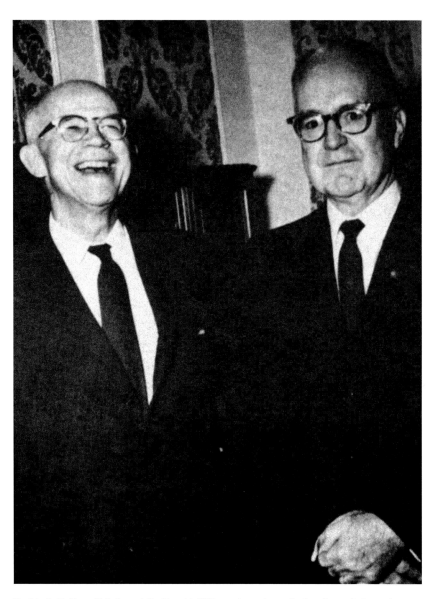

Dr. Mark R. Everett, left, and Dr. Don H. O'Donoghue at a 1963 faculty party honoring Dean Everett. *Courtesy University of Oklahoma.*

realized a new approach would be needed. The cart was before the horse. Before new doctors and nurses could be trained, basic science educational facilities were needed.

In September, 1964, Dennis met with Lester Gorsline, a California medical facilities planner, who would prove helpful in planning how to spend the $7 million proposed to expand the Medical Center. Dennis was able to interest Gorsline in his concept of sharing costs, facilities, space, and services with other entities to create a unified community health center rather than continue with the old idea of having just a medical school and an adjacent hospital.

Dennis was aware that a comprehensive health care campus could not be built without leadership from the power centers in Oklahoma City. It was no secret that publisher E.K. Gaylord had great influence. There were other groups of influence headed by bankers C.A. "Chuck" Vose and Harvey P. Everest. With Stanton L. Young, only in his thirties at the time and building bridges among leaders, the Oklahoma City business leadership firmly announced its support for the idea.

To create a master plan for an expanded medical center, Dennis appointed a planning committee headed by Dr. Bob Bird. Other members of the committee included Dr. Oren Skouge, director of the Veterans Administration Hospital (VA Hospital); Joe White, associate dean of the medical school; microbiologists Dr. Vernon Scott and Dr. Robert Patnode; University Hospital Administrator Raymond Crews; and OMRF President Leonard Eliel. Both the VA Hospital and OMRF were located in the Medical Center area on Northeast 13th Street close to University Hospital, Children's Hospital, and the medical school.

Dennis began meeting with civic leaders such as Stanton L. Young. They envisioned the new campus as a large, multi-

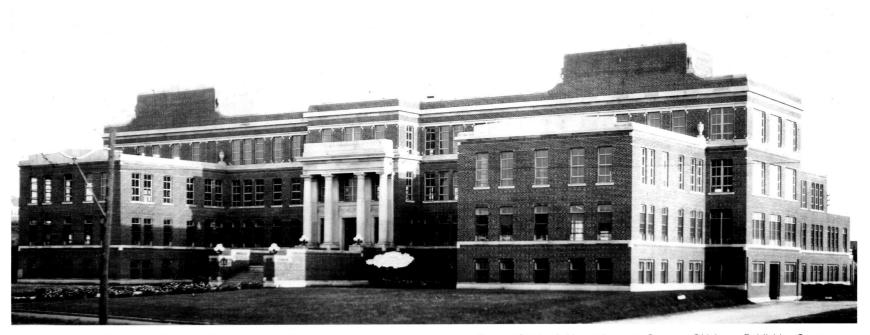

The nucleus of the Oklahoma City Medical Center—the medical school, University Hospital, and the Crippled Children's Hospital in 1935. *Courtesy Oklahoma Publishing Company.*

institutional center in which the federal and state governments would join with private health institutions and companies to assist OU's teaching mission by providing the practical, clinical experience health professionals would need to acquire their particular skills.

Working with the State Regents for Higher Education Chancellor E.T. Dunlap and his staff, Dennis recognized the benefit of the master plan being more than a plan for a medical center. It had to address the health concerns of the entire state. Dunlap believed Dennis' vision to help all of Oklahoma would sit well with the state legislature dominated by rural interests. It was not enough to improve health care only in the state's capital city. The legislature would become interested only if every section of the state could benefit by increased expenditures on Northeast 13th Street.

The State Regents for Higher Education appointed a blue-

ribbon citizens committee to advise them on state government's role in expansion of the Medical Center. Attorney John Rogers was chairman and Dean McGee was vice chairman. Henry Bellmon, Oklahoma's first Republican governor, had been in office less than two years when Dennis began selling his idea for a master plan for the Medical Center.

The citizens committee quickly found support for producing more doctors and nurses to remedy the shortage. Only 36 percent of the doctors in Oklahoma were in family practice and towns of fewer than 5,000 people had lost 135 doctors. The ratio of doctors to people in state was 115 per 100,000, far short of the national average of 151 physicians per 100,000 people. The Oklahoma Employment Security Commission suggested that double the number of registered nurses would be needed in the next 10 years.

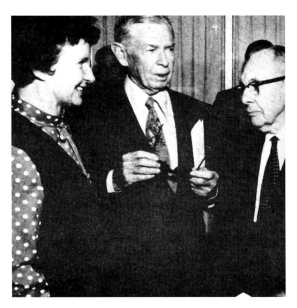

Early supporters of the Oklahoma Health Center complex, left to right, are Oklahoma City Mayor Patience Latting, banker Harvey P. Everest, and Tulsa attorney John Rogers. *Courtesy Oklahoma Heritage Association.*

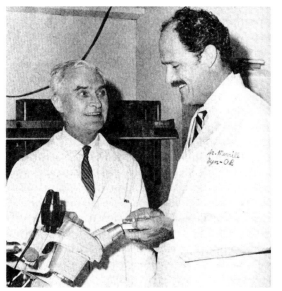

OU College of Medicine Dean Robert M. Bird and Gynecology-Obstetrics Chief James Merrill. *Courtesy University of Oklahoma.*

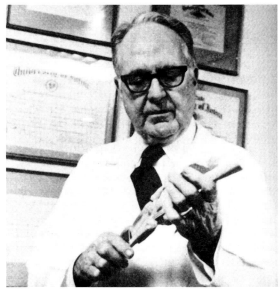

Dr. Don O'Donoghue was an orthopedist and sports medicine specialist. His belief in the campus approach for the Oklahoma Health Center never wavered. *Courtesy University of Oklahoma.*

There was much catching up to do. The need was obvious—the challenge was great.

Dennis first met McGee at a meeting at the offices of the Oklahoma City Chamber of Commerce set up by Stanley Draper and Stanton L. Young. Draper was a dedicated civic leader with a desire to do everything in his power to spur the Medical Center area growth. He had his finger on the pulse of important projects that impacted Oklahoma City. He tabbed Young as a future leader because of his involvement in the campaign of United States Senator Fred Harris.

At a subsequent meeting, McGee, William T. "Bill" Payne of Big Chief Drilling, E.K. Gaylord, and John Kirkpatrick agreed to accompany Dr. Dennis and Stanton L. Young on a tour of the Texas Medical Center (TMC) in Houston. Dennis believed that

TMC was a prototype of the kind of development he had in mind. McGee, Payne, Gaylord, and Kirkpatrick were joined on the tour by bankers Vose and Everest.

On the return trip home, Dennis could feel the adrenalin flowing. He later recalled, "For the first time, I think all these great community leaders felt it was a concept that was not just pie in the sky." Young, reflecting on the trip more than 40 years later, said, "There was electricity in the air as we talked about the possibilities. Everything was set up perfectly to capture a great opportunity in the life of Oklahoma."

It was fortuitous that McGee was a close friend of President Lyndon Johnson and served on a federal commission charged with increasing the number of medical graduates in the United States. McGee, with his contacts, was instrumental in helping Oklahoma

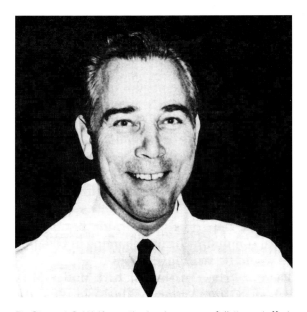

Dr. Stewart G. Wolf was the leader among full-time staff at the medical school in the early 1960s. *Courtesy University of Oklahoma.*

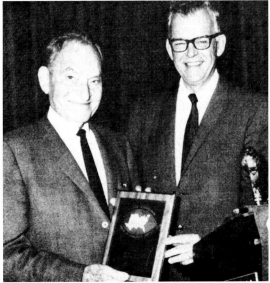

Stanley Draper, left, and Paul Strasbaugh were officials of the Oklahoma City Chamber of Commerce who were strong supporters of the development of the Oklahoma Health Center. *Courtesy Oklahoma Heritage Association.*

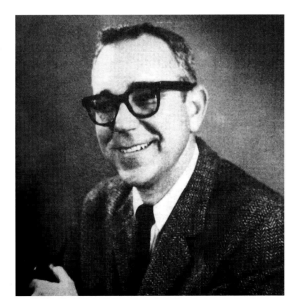

Dr. Joe White was chief of anesthesiology and associate dean of the OU College of Medicine. *Courtesy University of Oklahoma.*

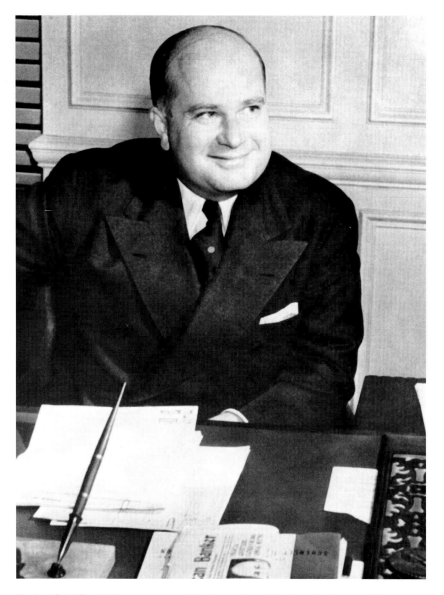

Banker C.A. "Chuck" Vose was an original supporter of the idea that became the Oklahoma Health Center. *Courtesy Oklahoma Publishing Company.*

learn how to submit proper applications for federal matching funds.

Dennis' idea of clustering more health organizations on a single campus was not without opposition. Some suspected it was an effort to centralize medical care in Oklahoma City rather than to provide convenient and comprehensive clinical experience for students learning to take care of the sick.

To sell his idea, Dennis needed participation of other health institutions. He also needed nearly $200 million to put his dream campus together. Leaders of OMRF and the VA Hospital were on board, so Dennis began talking to leaders of private Oklahoma City hospitals and directors of state and local government agencies.

Physicians at Presbyterian Hospital narrowly favored the idea of moving to the Medical Center area, even though board chairman Stanton L. Young was a leading proponent of the idea. Sister Mary Coletta, administrator of Mercy Hospital located two blocks west of Presbyterian Hospital, also expressed interest in moving to the Medical Center. However, the medical staff at Mercy opposed the move and was said to be looking for a location outside downtown Oklahoma City to build a new hospital. There was no doubt Mercy had to have new facilities. The original 25-bed section of the hospital was 49 years old, although the Sisters of Mercy had added another 200 beds after it purchased the hospital in 1947.

The Oklahoma State Department of Health was housed in an old Union Civil War soldiers' home at 3400 North Eastern Avenue and had outgrown its facilities. Commissioner of Health Dr. Kirk Mosley was excited about the possibility of moving to the Medical Center.

The Oklahoma City-County Health Department was scattered in four different buildings around the city. For a decade, Dr. M.L. Peter, the director, had been trying to secure a new building and wanted to be close to the Medical Center. There also was an effort by Dr. Richard Clay, an ophthalmologist, to develop an eye institute. In 1965, doctors and other citizens formed the Oklahoma Eye Foundation, a non-profit organization to set up an eye institute separate from Presbyterian Hospital.

Other elements had to fall in place to make possible a multi-institutional health campus. The Oklahoma City Urban Renewal Authority had designated areas around the proposed medical center as "renewal" areas, assuring affordable, federally-subsidized land for expansion. The Medical Center Urban Renewal Project was bound by Northeast 13th Street, Stonewall Avenue, Northeast 4th Street, and Durland Avenue, later named Lincoln Boulevard.

In the "renewal" area, Dr. Dennis could see an expanded horizon to the south, east, and west. He had the land, but faced unhappy residents in the area who would be removed from their longtime homes in order for the Medical Center to expand.

At a March 2, 1966 dinner meeting, hosted by Dean McGee and presided over by Governor Bellmon, the Oklahoma Health Sciences Foundation, now known as the Oklahoma Health Center Foundation (OHCF) was born. Its purpose was to expand the OU Medical Center into a comprehensive health sciences complex. The formation of the foundation was the first step in long-range planning for developing what supporters believed to be a $100-million complex to be called the Oklahoma Health Center (OHC).

Most of the trustees invited to the meeting heard Dr. Dennis explain his vision of at least 34 structures to accommodate hospitals, government agencies, research facilities, and teaching space. He emphasized the economic advantages of sharing centralized services such as a power plant and other behind-the-scenes operations. At the time, only Presbyterian Hospital and the Oklahoma Department of Health were committed to moving to the area. Robert C. Hardy, the

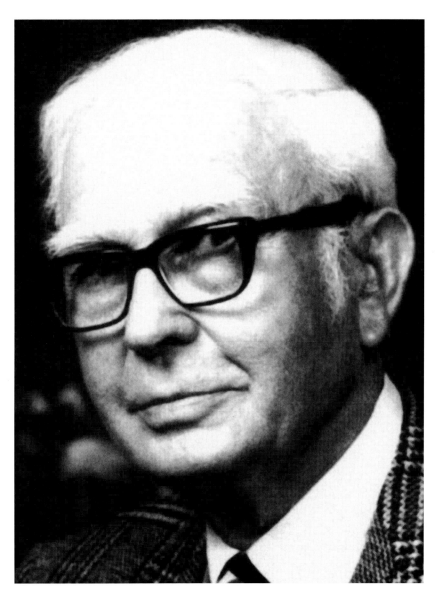

William T. Payne was a strong supporter of a comprehensive campus for the Oklahoma Health Center. *Courtesy Oklahoma Publishing Company.*

Original Incorporators of the Oklahoma Health Sciences Foundation

administrator of the University of Arkansas Hospital in Little Rock, was hired as the Foundation's director.

The creation of the Oklahoma Health Center brought a new era of medical services cooperation. Hospitals were being invited to sit at the same table with clinical teaching affiliates of the OU College of Medicine—together planning their future. They also were asked to help create and share centralized facilities to curb the rapidly rising cost of health care.

Lester Gorsline Associates was hired to coordinate the planning process. The Foundation's goal was to be the conduit through which each institution could carry out its primary role of patient care, research, teaching, or public health.

By March, 1967, Dr. Dennis and Lawrence Lackey, an architect and campus planner working with Gorsline, presented revised plans for the Oklahoma Health Center. The plans laid out essential facilities on a 176-acre site to the west, south, and east of the existing 24-acre Medical Center.

That same month, the Oklahoma Regents for Higher Education asked the Oklahoma legislature for more than $40 million to expand and improve the Medical Center. Senator Bryce Baggett, whose district included the Medical Center area, introduced a resolution calling for a $47 million state bond issue to expand the Medical Center and construct a new building for the Oklahoma Department of Health. However, the bond issue was delayed.

Oklahoma's new governor, Dewey Bartlett, would not support the call for the bond issue until he could gain additional information. He appointed a citizen's expenditure advisory council, chaired by Dean McGee, to work with Baggett and the State Regents. Other members of the advisory council included Stanton L. Young, John Rogers of Tulsa, and William D. Little of Ada.

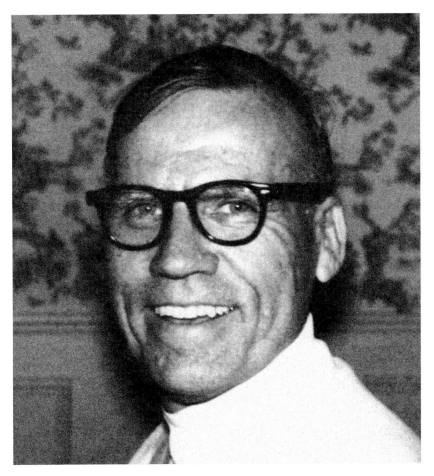

With 20 years experience in hospital planning and administration, Robert Hardy was the first executive director of the Oklahoma Health Sciences Foundation. *Courtesy Oklahoma Health Center Foundation.*

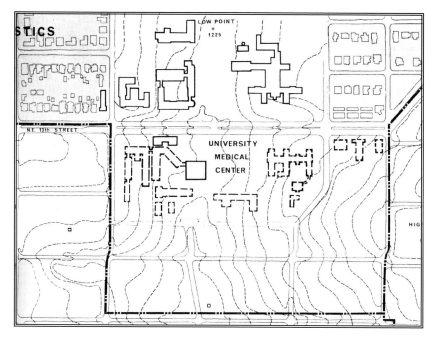

The land that was proposed for the expansion of the Oklahoma Health Center was located in two areas designated by the Oklahoma City Urban Renewal Authority. The plan called for the removal of buildings to make way for construction of new facilities for tenants of OHC. *Courtesy Oklahoma Health Center Foundation.*

Dr. Bob Bird and his planning committee continued to prepare applications for federal grants with the hope bond money would be forthcoming. In early 1968, the formal plan for the Oklahoma Health Center was published. The plan proposed 14 institutions to be involved, plus a residential development for 1,000 students. It was estimated 28,000 students, staff, visitors, and outpatients would visit the campus each week. There was planning for more than 10,000 parking spaces.

Based upon recommendations of Governor Bartlett's study committee, the Oklahoma legislature approved a $99.8 million bond issue to be submitted to state voters. The bond issue was called Health and Education for a Richer Oklahoma (HERO). From the money, legislators proposed the Medical Center receive more than $26 million and the State Health Department receive $4.5 million for its new building.

Dr. Dennis had succeeded in convincing legislators it was impossible to build a huge hospital in every city and town in Oklahoma, but a world-class medical complex could provide personnel and support services to supplement medical care provided in the local community. At the time, Senator Baggett said, "Dr. Dennis developed a receptive mood on the part of the legislators to recognize that the large, central facility operated by the University of Oklahoma was critical to their home town interest."

Strongly supported by the chambers of commerce in Tulsa and Oklahoma City, the HERO bond issue had something for everyone, including projects in several college and university towns. The money raised from the sale of the bonds would be repaid by a five-cent increase on each pack of cigarettes sold in the state. Supporters reasoned that the increased health risk of smokers justified their paying the bill for expanded medical facilities in Oklahoma.

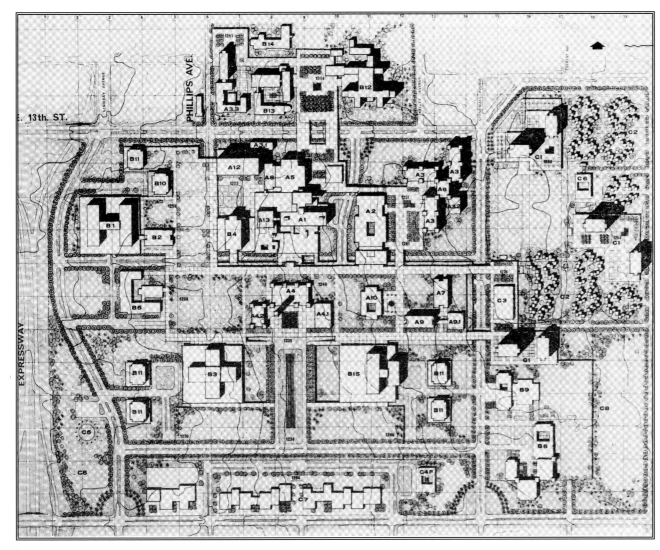

Schematic Plan for the Oklahoma Health Center— January 1967

A1   University Teaching Hospital
A2   Basic Sciences Teaching
A3   Research, Basic Sciences
A3.1 Existing Medical Research
A3.2 Dentistry Research
A3.3 Graduate College
A4   Library, Computer Facilities
A4.1 Auditorium, Continuing Education
A4.2 OHSF Administration,
      Medical Center Administration,
      Health Education Services Center
A5   OPD, Medical
A6   Central Animal Facilities
A7   University School of Nursing
A8   OPD, Dentistry
A9   School of Public Health
A9.1 School of Allied Health Sciences
A10 Student Union
A12 University Mental Health Complex
A13 Rehabilitation and Chronic Disease Wing
B1   Presbyterian Hospital
B2   Mercy Hospital
B4   Children's Hospital
B5   Community Mental Health Center
B8   State Department of Public Health
B9   Oklahoma City–County Health Department
B10 Oklahoma City Clinic
B11 Other Clinics
B12 Veterans Administration Hospital
B13 Oklahoma Medical Research Foundation
B14 Speech and Hearng Center
B15 Hospital
C1   Student Residence Facilities—High Rise
C2   Student Residence Facilities—Low Rise
C3   Indoor Health and Recreation Facilities
C4   Central Services
C4C Heating Plant
C4F Preschool Nursery
C5   Heliport
C6   University Elementary Laboratory School
C7   Neighborhood Shops
C8   Reserve Area

The proposed plan for development of the Oklahoma Health Center as presented to the public in January, 1967. *Courtesy Oklahoma Health Center Foundation.*

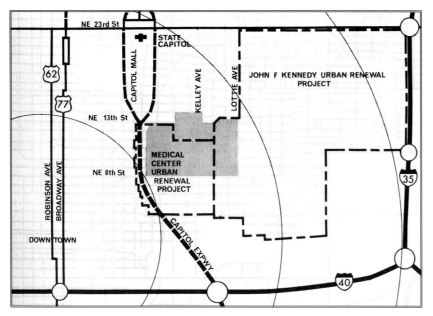

The proposed expressway south of the State Capitol to improve access to the emerging Oklahoma Health Center. *Courtesy Oklahoma Health Center Foundation.*

A massive public relations program was launched to convince voters to approve HERO. Dr. Dennis gave much of the credit for creating a positive image for OHC funding to OU College of Medicine alumni scattered throughout the state. *The Daily Oklahoman* published a series of articles in the weeks before the December 10, 1968 election.

The hard-hitting facts showed that Oklahoma needed 1,500 doctors, as many as 4,800 nurses, and at least 25,000 other health-related professionals. Voters were impressed with the argument and approved the bond issue by a 3 to 1 margin.

Even before the bond money became available, construction crews were hard at work expanding the Oklahoma Health Center. In 1967, the OU Foundation funded a $144,000 Family Medicine Clinic at Northeast 15th Street and Phillips Avenue, the first new building to be constructed in the health center. Ground was broken the same year for the Basic Sciences Education Building north of the old school of nursing. The building was primarily financed by a $2.1 million grant from the federal government. At the ground breaking, Dr. Dennis remarked, "This great health education venture is no longer a dream. It is happening!"

With HERO bond money available, planners began turning out new proposals. Educational programs were launched before there were facilities to house them. Space in 28 houses on Northeast 14th, 15th, and 16th streets between Lindsay and Lincoln boulevards was developed to accommodate dentistry, dental hygiene, public health, pharmacy, and many expanded administrative activities for the new center.

In June, 1969, the University of Oklahoma Board of Regents approved a $11.9 million bid to build the first 200 beds of the new University Hospital. The project was funded by HERO bonds,

Hill-Burton federal funds, and a grant from the federal Health Professions Educational Assistance Program.

In June, 1970, the Basic Sciences Education Building was dedicated, making it possible to increase the size of the entering class of medical school from 104 to 126. OU created an office of architectural and engineering services to coordinate plans for construction and develop long-range plans to fit into leaders' dreams for the entire Oklahoma Health Center. Arthur Tuttle, Jr. was the first director of the department and immediately began working on the proposed School of Dentistry, the School of Public Health, and the Health Sciences Library.

Dr. Mark Allen Everett, son of the former dean of the College of Medicine and vice president for health sciences, was chairman of the Department of Dermatology. Everett planned, financed, and built the Dermatology Clinic on Northeast 13th Street as a separate facility.

Even more important to the success of the Oklahoma Health Center than building facilities was recruitment of excellent faculty. Stanton L. Young remembered, "It was great to see construction in the area, but OHC would never have achieved its desired level of success without the hiring of outstanding administrators and faculty members who brought both prestige and federal research dollars to the center."

Joining the acknowledged leader of the emerging full-time faculty at the medical school, Dr. Stewart G. Wolf, were Dr. Mark Allen Everett, Dr. John Schilling, Dr. Bill Thurman, Dr. Eleanor Knudsen, Dr. Tom Points, Dr. John Bruhn, Dr. G. Rainey Williams, Dr. Bill Stanhope, Dr. Bill Schottstaedt, and Dr. Bill Brown, who was charged with building a dental college from scratch.

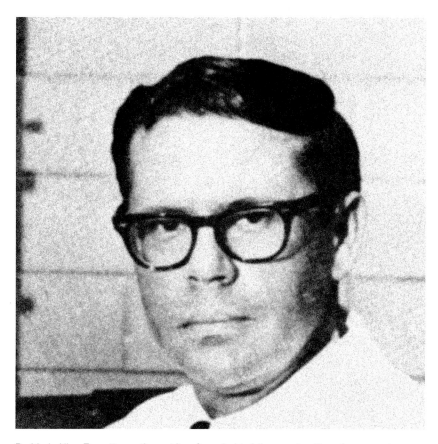

Dr. Mark Allen Everett was the guiding force behind the construction of a separate Dermatology Clinic. *Courtesy University of Oklahoma.*

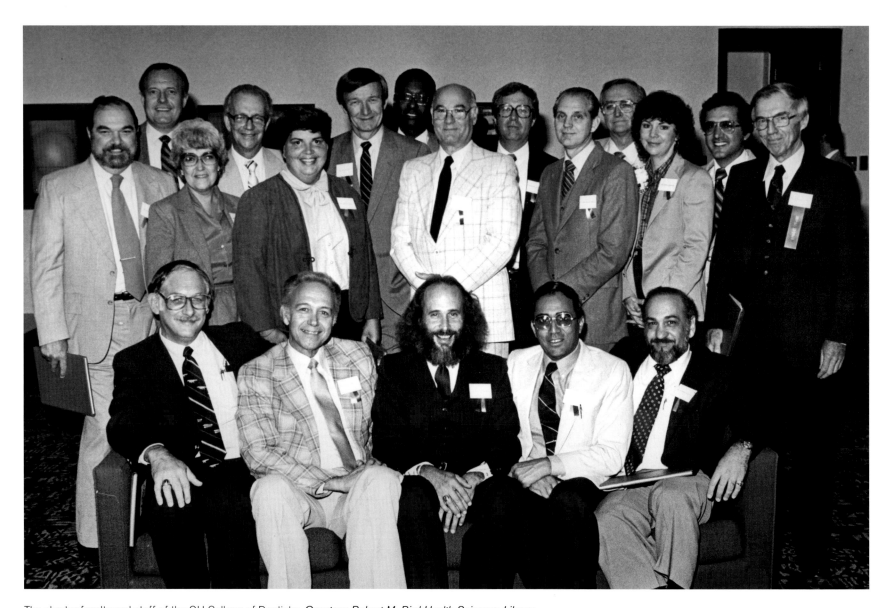

The charter faculty and staff of the OU College of Dentistry. *Courtesy Robert M. Bird Health Sciences Library.*

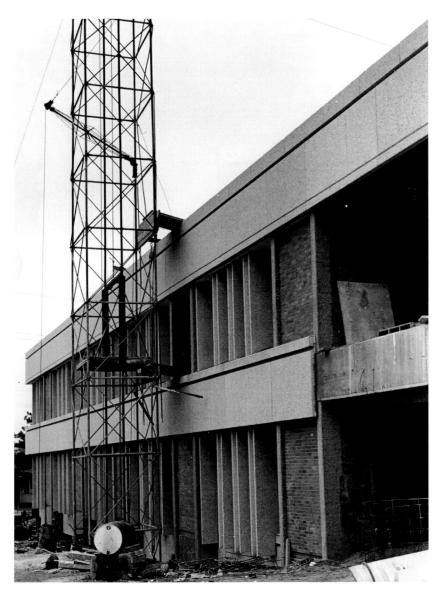

Contractors put the finishing touches on the Basic Sciences Education Building in 1969.
Courtesy Oklahoma Publishing Company.

The Lackey Plan

California campus planner Lawrence Lackey developed the original plans for the Medical Center in 1968. Lackey's idea envisioned a true campus with buildings well spaced, the areas between them attractively landscaped, and wide boulevards providing for easy vehicle access and circulation. A unifying feature of the campus was a parking "blanket" that followed the contour of the land. The parking provided two levels for the protection of parked cars and a landscaped top for pedestrians with connecting bridges to major buildings. Lackey theorized that all automobiles would be "indoors" and the campus would retain a pleasing environment and not become one vast, continuous used car lot.

When it was determined that the parking structures could not be funded, the underlying concepts of the Lackey Plan were reconsidered and important departures were outlined. Some of the functional relationships of the major elements of the plan were maintained. The present arrangement of buildings emerged from years of discussions among the Oklahoma Health Sciences Foundation, now the Oklahoma Health Center Foundation; the Oklahoma City Urban Renewal Authority; and the University of Oklahoma Health Sciences Center. The "master plan" always has been a "plan in progress" as new buildings were authorized, designed, and constructed.

Chapter Three

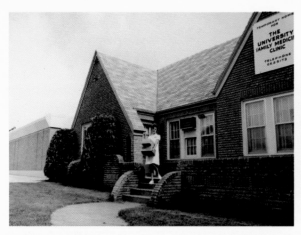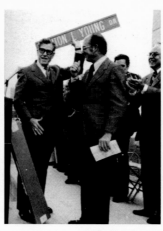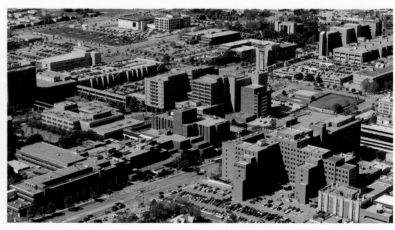

Difficult Times

While the HERO bond issue perhaps solved the need for construction capital to match federal grants, the Medical Center began running short of operating funds. The state legislature was increasing appropriations for operations at the rate of five or six percent per year, but rising costs were exceeding 20 percent annually. During the late 1960s, the cost per patient per day at University Hospital increased from $28 to $63.

Other problems arose.

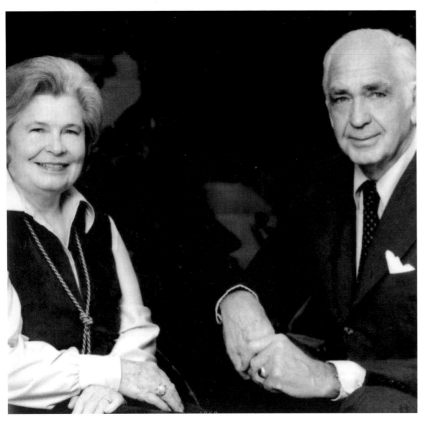

Eleanor and John Kirkpatrick took an active interest in the move of Presbyterian Hospital to the Oklahoma Health Center. Kirkpatrick was a successful oil man. He and his wife were generous philanthropists. *Courtesy Oklahoma Publishing Company.*

The doctors who ran Mercy Hospital overruled the wishes of Sister Mary Coletta, who had publicly announced that Mercy should become a teaching hospital affiliated with OU. Instead, at least half the doctors who practiced at Mercy wanted to move to northwest Oklahoma City. In early 1970, it was announced that the new Mercy Hospital would be built on a 40-acre site at Meridian Avenue and Memorial Road.

Another difficulty was the relationship between Governor Bartlett and J. Herbert Holloman, who had succeeded George L. Cross as president of OU. Dr. Holloman's management style also concerned Dr. Dennis. When Dennis believed he could no longer work with Holloman, he resigned on July 7, 1970, and returned to Arkansas as chancellor of the University of Arkansas Medical Center in Little Rock. Less than three weeks later, Holloman resigned.

In addition to university expansion, Presbyterian Hospital officials announced in September, 1970, that it was buying 24 acres, an L-shaped parcel of land between Durland Avenue, now Lincoln Boulevard, and Phillips Avenue. The hospital paid only $300,000 for the land. Plans were announced to build a $23 million hospital. Four years later, when the hospital opened, it cost $37 million. However, the hospital became an integral part of OHC.

It was a critical time in the life of the Oklahoma Health Center. Replacing Dr. Dennis, Dr. John Colmore became acting vice president of OU for medical affairs, but died two months later. Dr. Len Eliel replaced Dr. Colmore and faced immediate funding problems that hampered the implementation of Dr. Dennis' dreams.

Dr. William D. "Bill" Stanhope was hired to organize an educational program for physicians' associates. The program was directed to alleviate the growing healthcare shortage in rural Oklahoma. A help to increase the number of trained healthcare

(Facing page) A vacant house and an oil derrick were the last remnants of the past removed from the corner of Northeast 13th Street and Lindsay Avenue to make way for construction of the new Presbyterian Hospital. *Courtesy Oklahoma Publishing Company.*

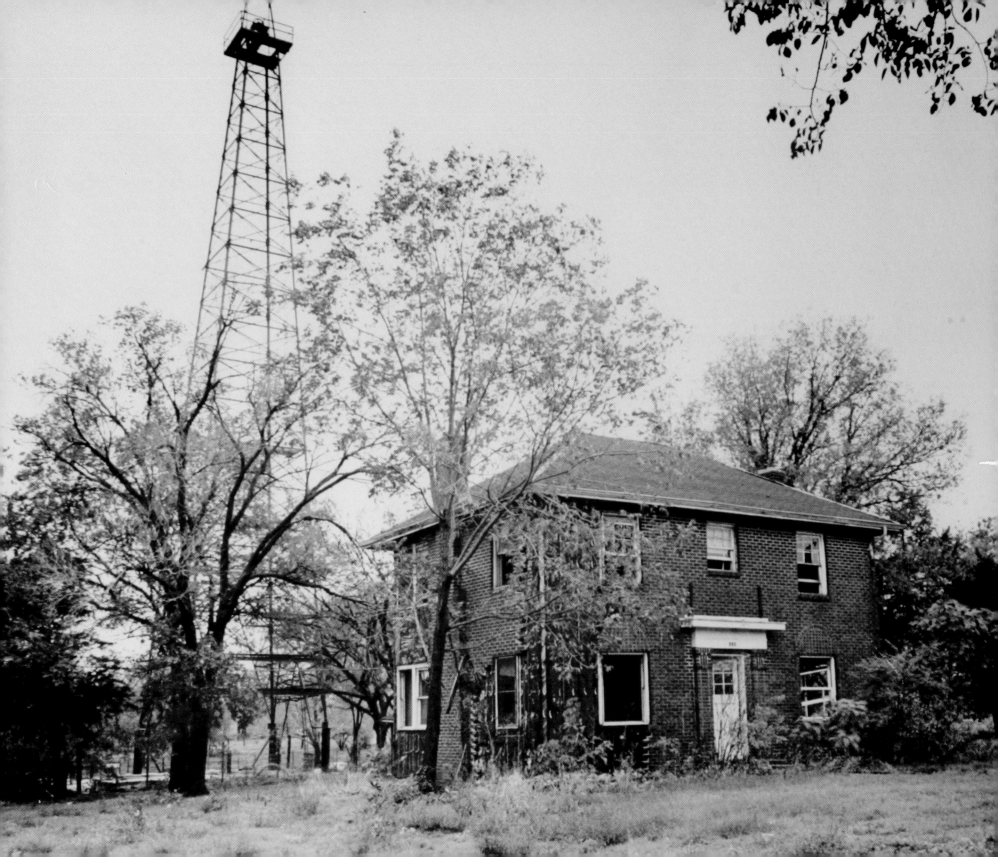

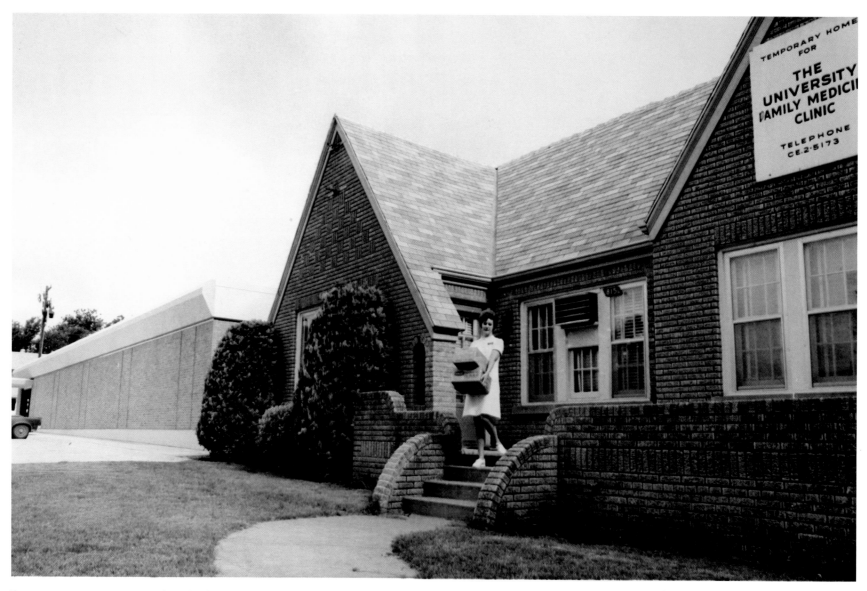

For many years, new programs of the OU College of Medicine and other OU professional schools were headquartered in aging houses in the surrounding neighborhood. In 1968, the new family medicine clinic opened in a house on North Phillips Avenue. *Courtesy Oklahoma Publishing Company.*

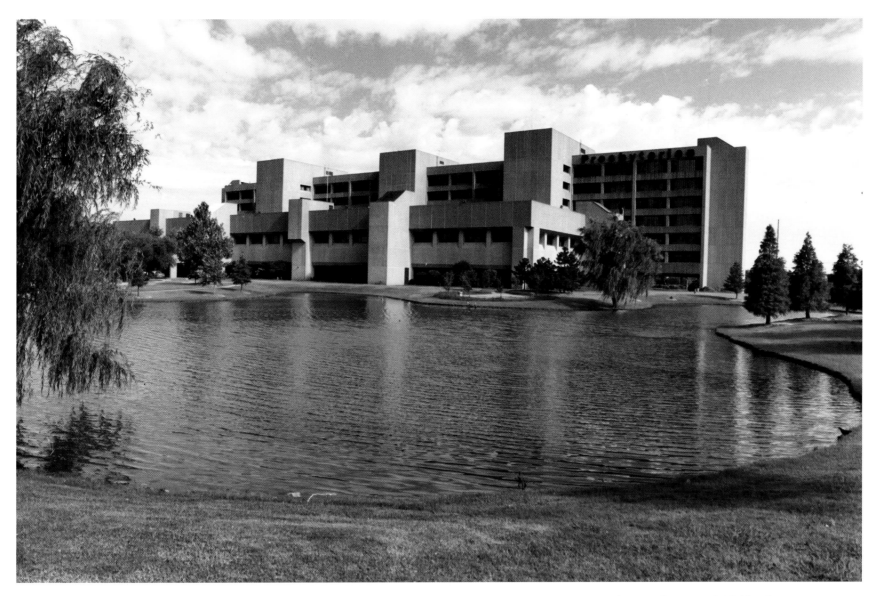

Presbyterian Hospital was the first major non-university facility to commit to relocating in the Oklahoma Health Center complex. *Courtesy Oklahoma Publishing Company.*

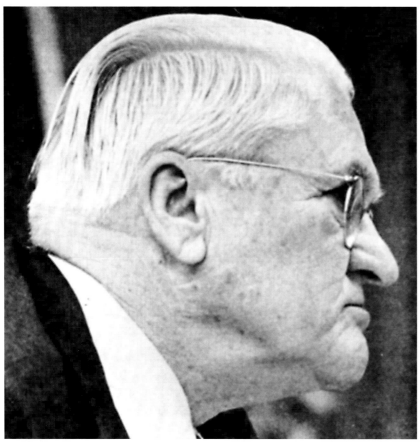

Lloyd Rader, as head of the Oklahoma Department of Welfare, now the Department of Human Services, wielded great influence in state government. He is credited with saving Children's Hospital and University Hospital. *Courtesy Department of Human Services.*

workers was talkback television, introduced on campus in 1971. The instruction system was designed to take the college classroom to industry and business in a dozen cities and towns throughout the state.

A strong supporter of increased state funding for OHC was Representative William P. "Bill" Willis of Tahlequah. Dr. Eliel sold Willis on the idea that the Medical Center's money problems could be solved if the state came up with $45 million. During the 1970s battles for increased funding, the name of the Medical Center was changed to the OU Health Sciences Center to better reflect the expanded role.

In February, 1971, Dr. William W. Schottstaedt, dean of the School of Health, announced a new $10 million building to house the school. Seventy percent of the cost of the project would be paid by the federal government. Dr. Leroy Carpenter became Oklahoma Commissioner of Health and assured the close association between the educational programs and public health.

In the summer of the 1971, the School of Health Related Professions, later Allied Health, began a four-year curriculum in dental hygiene in cooperation with the College of Dentistry. Temporary clinical facilities were set up in an old house at Northeast 14th Street and Lindsay Avenue.

In December, 1971, United States Senator Henry Bellmon announced that the federal Department of Health, Education, and Welfare had approved a $1.2 million grant for the construction of a third floor, a $1.8 million dental addition to the Basic Sciences Education Building matched with HERO bond money. However, as the grant was announced, it became public knowledge that federal funding was getting tight.

Before federal funds became less accessible, other OHC building projects began. The VA Hospital announced a $2 million research addition that added 30,000 square feet of laboratory space that allowed other space in the existing hospital to be used for patient care. The federal government was struggling nationwide to keep up with the demand for treatment of veterans at the nation's 166 VA hospitals.

In 1971, a $4 million steam and chilled water plant was dedicated, an important element of the idea of cost-sharing for buildings in the complex. Also in 1971, OMRF dedicated a new office building named for John Rogers, Tulsa attorney and civic leader. Plans progressed for obtaining funding for the Dental Clinical Sciences Building. A year later, $16.5 million in federal funds became available to match $5.5 million in HERO bonds to build the dental building and a building to house biomedical sciences and the library. The campus was beginning to take shape.

Overshadowing the good news of new infusion of building money for the campus was the fact that University Hospital was in trouble because it could not collect its bills from the increasing number of indigent patients. New OU President Paul Sharp was concerned that the state did not have sufficient financial means to pay the rising operational costs for all the services for which it had money to construct buildings. The money crisis at University included times when payroll was difficult to make. There was talk of closing Children's Hospital and moving its patients to Old Main.

Oklahoma's new governor, David Hall, also was concerned whether Oklahoma could afford the expansion underway. In 1964, the state appropriation for the Medical Center was $3.1 million, but had grown to $10.5 million by 1972, and was $2 million less than Dr. Eliel suggested was needed. The governor appointed attorney Robert E. Lee Richardson to conduct an independent investigation of the university-affiliated programs and teaching institutions on the Oklahoma City campus.

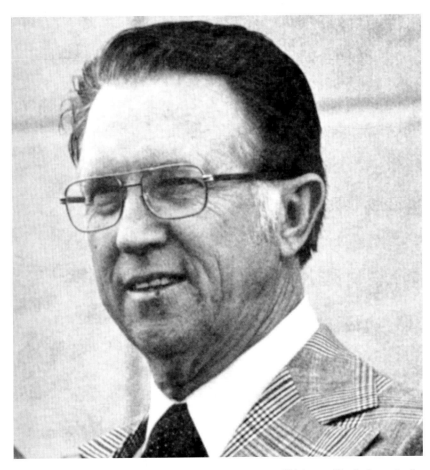

Dr. Richard Clay pioneered the idea for an eye institute in Oklahoma City that eventually became the Dean A. McGee Eye Institute. *Courtesy Oklahoma Publishing Company.*

Political, university, and city leaders looked closely at the crisis. A position paper produced by the Oklahoma City Chamber of Commerce in April, 1973, called the Medical Center's financial crunch a serious crisis and predicted that Oklahoma's future generations would not have high quality medical care if the health sciences education system was allowed to fail.

Student enrollment had doubled to 1,750 by 1973 and construction of the OHC concept was well underway. Community leaders urged the legislature to act promptly and decisively to solve the financial crisis. OU Regents requested $4.4 million in additional money to open the newly completed, 214-bed Mark Everett Tower at University Hospital.

After much political wrangling, the state legislature in 1973 transferred the operation of University Hospital from the OU Board of Regents to a new board of trustees and greatly increased funding.

The legislature also transferred control of Children's Hospital to the Oklahoma Department of Institutions, Social, and Rehabilitative Services, formerly the Oklahoma Department of Public Welfare. It was a major move for the university to give up control of its two hospitals, but financial and political conditions mandated such action.

Welfare Director Lloyd Rader hit the ground running with Children's Hospital, helped by a $1.3 million appropriation to remodel and expand the hospital. Even with the political and funding problems, the idea for a comprehensive Oklahoma Health Center was alive and well.

The disparity in funding for University Hospital and Children's Hospital was obvious. In 1974, the State Senate approved a $6.68 million appropriation to operate University, although administrators believed expenses would have to be cut $160,000 a month to break even.

A second wave of OHC leaders began to make a difference. William G. "Bill" Thurman became provost of the OU Health Sciences Center in 1975. Also, leaders of an effort to build a regional eye institute succeeded in bringing their dream to a reality. For a decade, the Oklahoma Eye Foundation, organized by Dr. Richard Clay, had struggled to raise money for construction of an eye institute. The struggle became easier when oilman Dean McGee suffered an eye problem.

McGee was scheduled for eye surgery in January, 1971, with Johns Hopkins-trained ophthalmologist Dr. Tullos Coston. While having his eye dressed after surgery, McGee casually asked Dr. Coston if good ophthalmology training was available in Oklahoma. When informed that Oklahoma did not have an institute at which quality training in the field could be provided, McGee replied, "You know, that might be arranged."

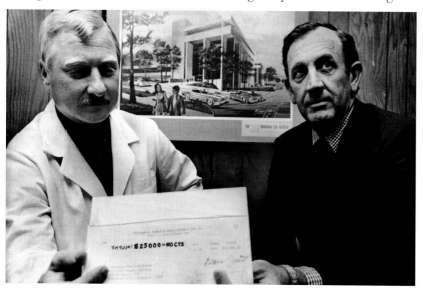

John March, right, of the Noble Foundation, presents Dr. Tom Acers, director of the Dean A. McGee Eye Institute, a check in 1974 to help construct the new eye institute building. *Courtesy Oklahoma Publishing Company.*

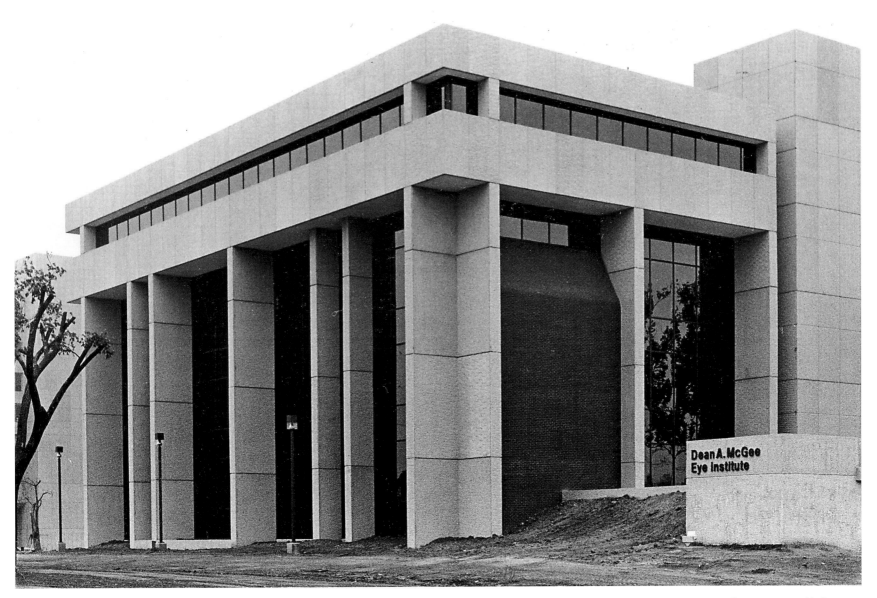

The Dean A. McGee Eye Institute nears completion in 1975. Oilman Dean A. McGee provided the impetus to help health care providers realize the dream of creating a world-class eye treatment and research site. *Courtesy Oklahoma Publishing Company.*

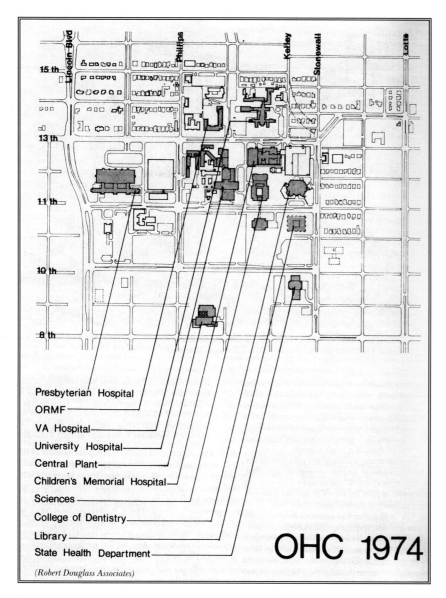

Presbyterian Hospital
ORMF
VA Hospital
University Hospital
Central Plant
Children's Memorial Hospital
Sciences
College of Dentistry
Library
State Health Department

OHC 1974

(Robert Douglass Associates)

The Oklahoma Health Center as it appeared in 1974 in an architect's drawing. *Courtesy Oklahoma Health Center Foundation.*

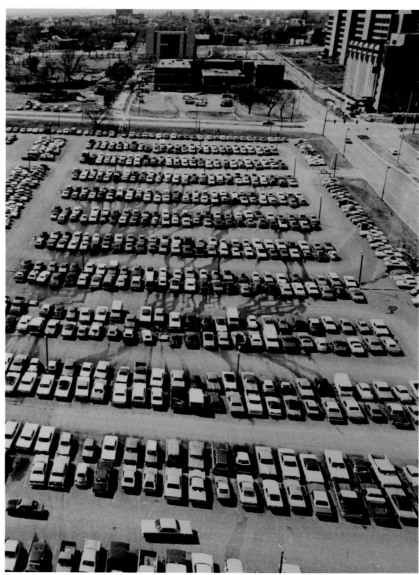

Before the addition of parking garages, a sea of cars parked in the central parking lot of the medical center campus in the 1970s. *Courtesy Oklahoma Publishing Company.*

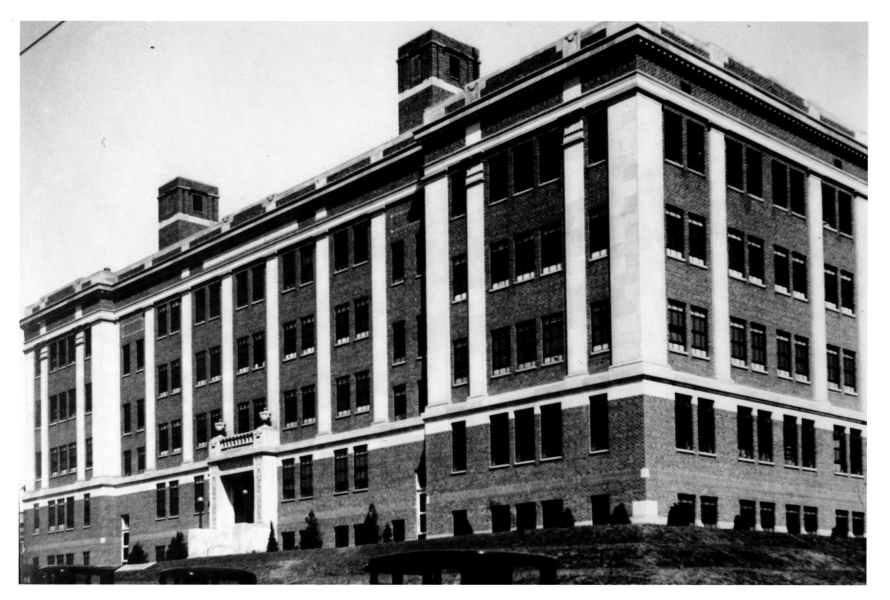

The OU College of Medicine had little room for expansion or laboratory experiments in its aged building. *Courtesy Oklahoma Publishing Company.*

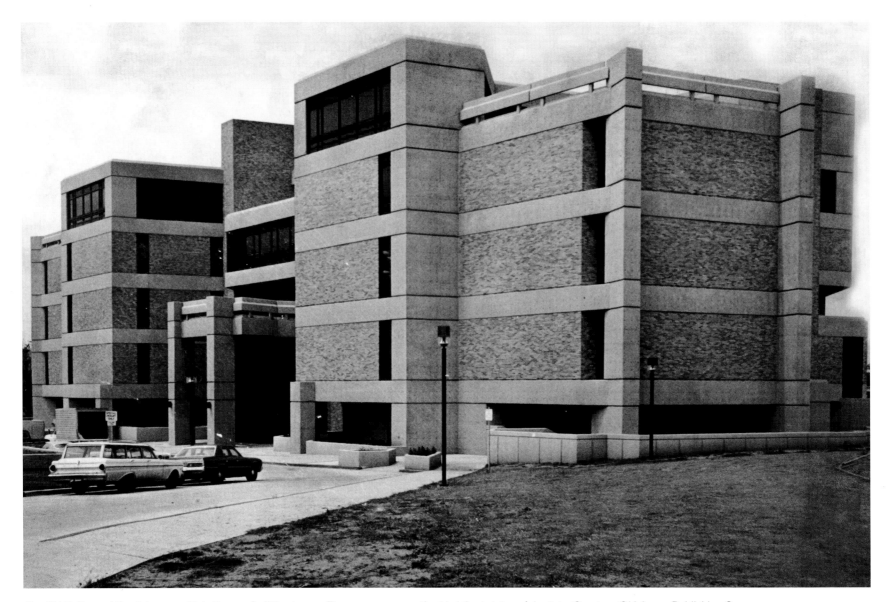

The OU College of Dentistry moved into its new facilities in 1977. The new space greatly aided the training of dentists. *Courtesy Oklahoma Publishing Company.*

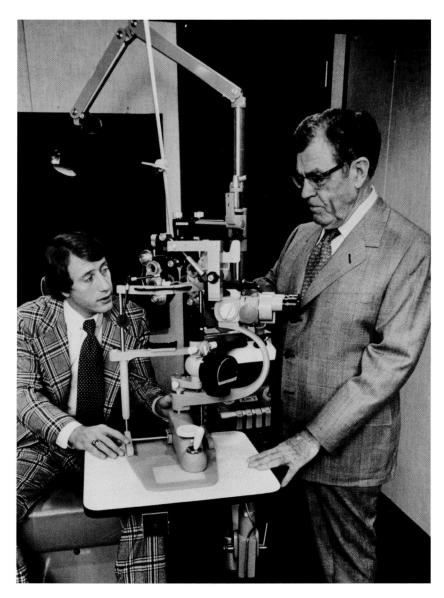

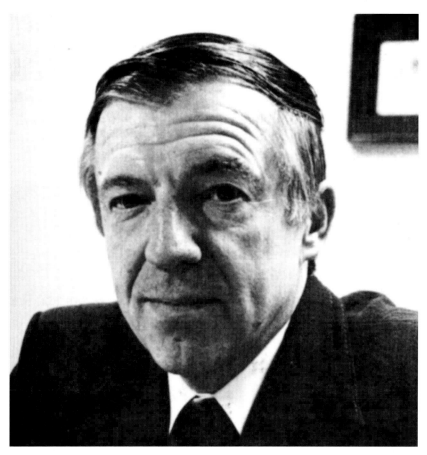

Dr. William "Bill" Brown took on the challenge of building a dental college on the campus of the Oklahoma Health Center from ground up. *Courtesy University of Oklahoma.*

In 1976, Dean A. McGee, right, and Cary Sully, look over equipment in an eye examination room at the Dean A. McGee Eye Institute. Sully was chairman of the annual Bachelors Club Christmas Ball which raised money for the eye institute. *Courtesy Oklahoma Publishing Company.*

With McGee's backing, the idea that became the Dean A. McGee Eye Institute moved forward. Stanton L. Young, E.K. Gaylord, and bankers Jack Conn and Chuck Vose began planning for a fundraising effort. In December, 1975, the institute opened for patient services. As part of the dedication of the new facility, the four-block portion of Northeast 11th Street was renamed Stanton L. Young Boulevard, in honor of the man who contributed so much time and effort to make possible the expansion of the OHC campus.

Belt-tightening by the federal government in the administration of President Richard Nixon caused Welfare Director Rader to abandon plans to build a new Children's Hospital. Instead, Rader obtained federal and state funds to continue expanding the old building on every side. By 1976, a new nursing tower, named for veteran pediatrician, George H. Garrison, was completed.

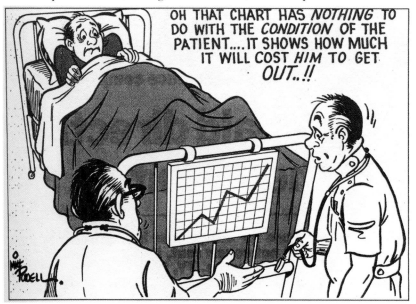

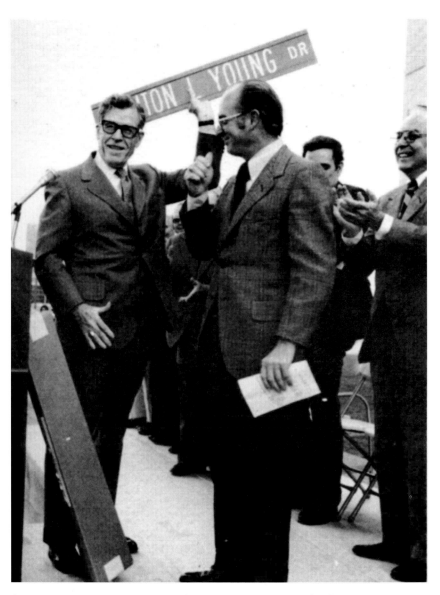

The Daily Oklahoman featured a cartoon titled "The High Cost of Being Sick" that explained the alarming rise of medical costs in the United States. *Courtesy Oklahoma Publishing Company.*

Stanton L. Young smiles as Dean McGee holds up the new sign for Stanton L. Young Boulevard. The boulevard runs through the center of the Oklahoma Health Center campus. *Courtesy Oklahoma Publishing Company.*

(Facing page) An modern view of the Oklahoma Health Center campus. *Courtesy Oklahoma Publishing Company.*

44

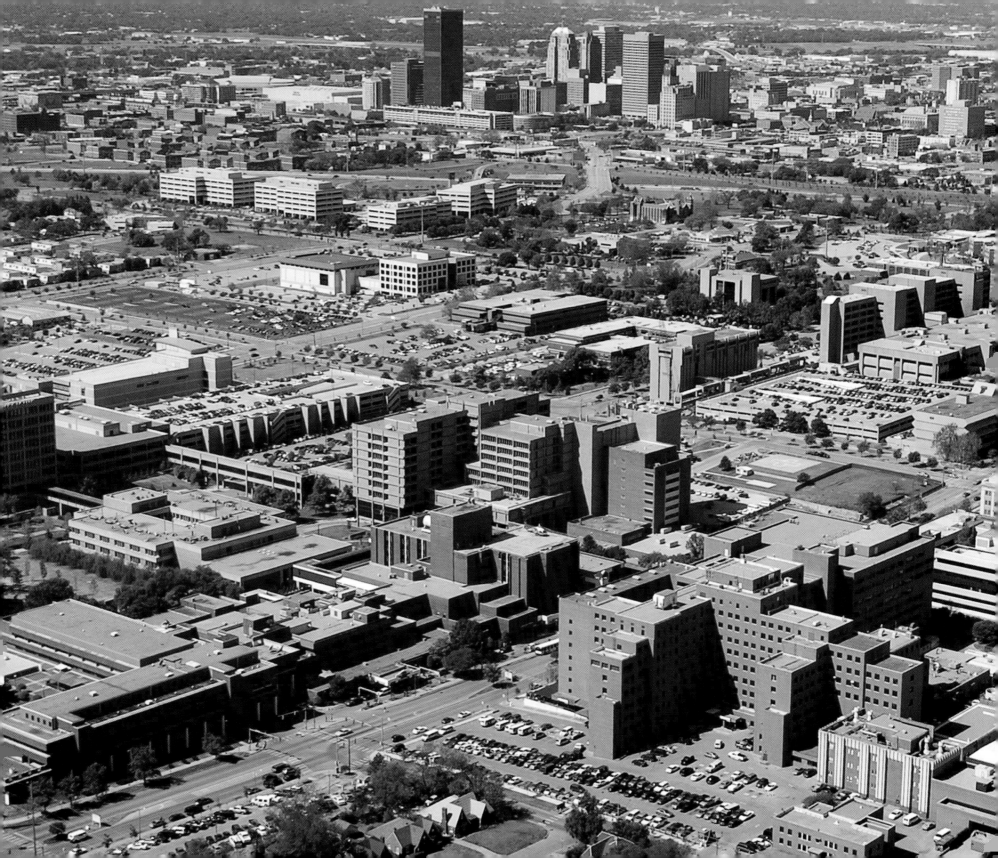

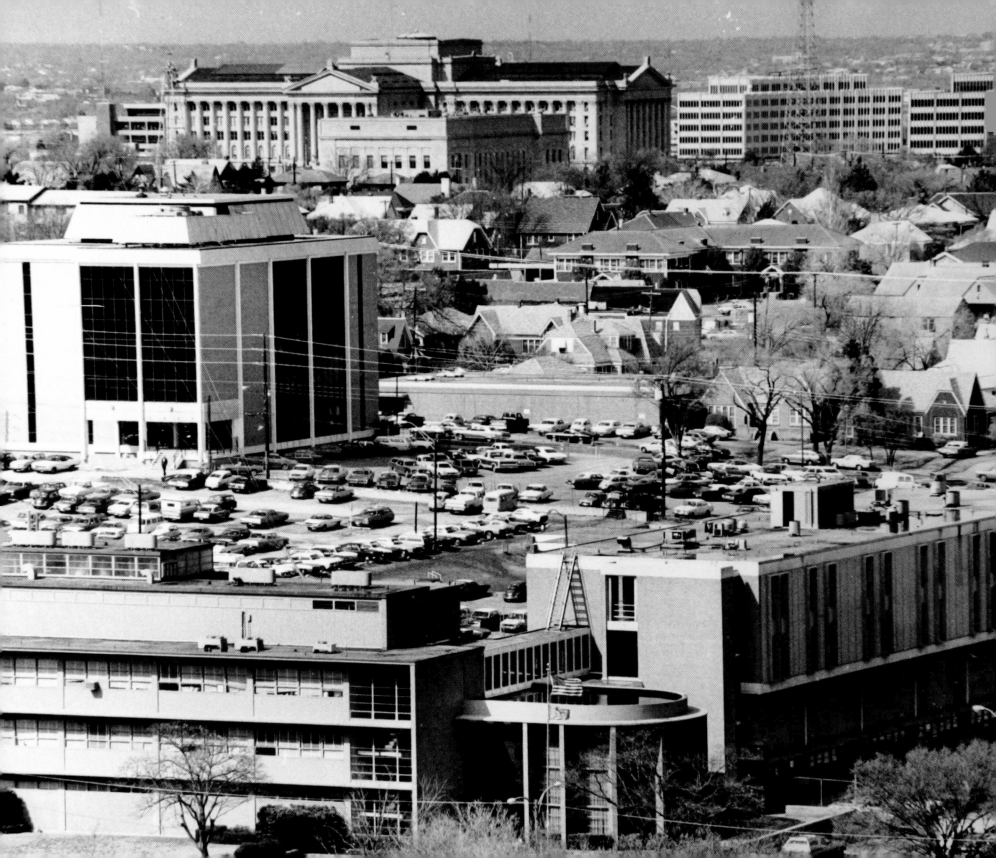

Rader also attracted top quality physicians and administrators. Dr. Donald B. Halverstadt became chief of staff at Children's Hospital. Dr. Mark Allen Everett became chief of staff at University Hospital.

Even with major advances in creating a campus, there was still a cluster of "camping out" in old houses for many programs. When the OU College of Pharmacy moved from the Norman campus to Oklahoma City in 1976, Dean Rodney Ice was faced with training pharmacists in seven different houses. Dean Ice's problem was similar to that of other program directors. Ice said, "When you are scattered, you have problems with maintaining identity. It's hard to bring everyone together. It's hard to have unity in purpose."

The Dental Clinical Services Building was dedicated in April, 1976. In October of that year, the $11 million, ten-story Biomedical Sciences Building opened. The building was designed primarily to accommodate offices and research laboratories of the basic science faculty.

The enrollment of the College of Nursing had grown to 335 students by the time the College of Nursing Building was ready for occupancy in July, 1977. Dean Gloria Smith believed the new four-story, 93,000 square foot building changed the image of nursing in Oklahoma.

By the spring of 1978, the shells of the fourth and fifth floors of the Dean A. McGee Eye Institute were completed. The fourth floor was dedicated to eye research, made possible by a $2 million gift from Cora Snetcher. The expansion, not visible from the outside, was a major advance in ophthalmology and came just two years after the institute opened.

It was an active spring and summer in 1978 for OHC openings. In June, the Oklahoma Medical Research Foundation held an open house for its newly-expanded building. Research patients were moved to Presbyterian Hospital, making space available for administrative and research functions, and a 20,000 square foot wing was added.

(Left) A view of the Oklahoma Medical Research Foundation in foreground from the top of the Biomedical Sciences Building in 1976. *Courtesy Oklahoma Publishing Company.*

In July, the 50 physicians of the Oklahoma City Clinic moved into a new, two-story building at Northeast 10th Street and Phillips Avenue. The clinic was the first group practice established in Oklahoma, founded in 1919 by six physicians who were dedicated to providing quality healthcare. The doctors had provided staffing for Wesley Hospital for years and maintained a general practice for the community along with their interest in teaching.

At first, there was resistance to moving the clinic to the OHC area. However, once the new Presbyterian Hospital's mission was clear, leaders of the Oklahoma City Clinic, including Dr. Jack Records, moved swiftly to raise the money to build a new building in the Medical Center area.

The new Oklahoma City Clinic offered family medicine, internal medical, pediatrics, and other disciplines. The clinic also featured a full service radiology center, laboratory, and pharmacy.

In August, 1978, it took three weeks to move books and journals from the old medical school building into the new Robert M. Bird Health Sciences Library at Stonewall Avenue and Stanton L. Young Boulevard. The four-level facility was the heart of the campus and was in the geographic center of the colleges.

In the same month, the new State Medical Examiner's Office building was occupied at Stonewall Avenue and Northeast 8th Street. Construction also began on a 1,100 space, $3.7 million parking structure for the university.

At about the same time the Oklahoma City Clinic was moving to the health campus, the eight doctors who made up the Oklahoma Allergy Clinic considered relocating. Founded in 1925 as the Balyeat Hay Fever and Asthma Clinic, after its founder, Dr. Ray Balyeat, the practice was highly respected in allergy and asthma diagnostic, treatment, and research.

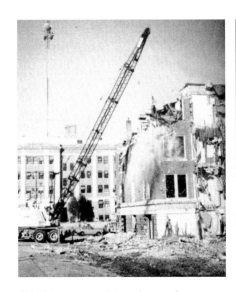

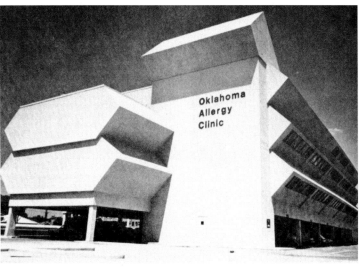

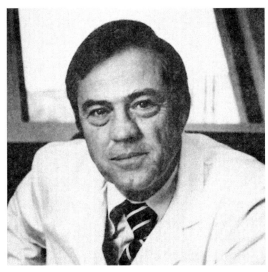

Old Main was razed to make way for new construction on the Oklahoma Health Center campus. As programs expanded, older buildings were leveled and new buildings were built. *Courtesy University of Oklahoma.*

The new Oklahoma Allergy Clinic Building opened on the Oklahoma Health Center campus in 1977. *Courtesy University of Oklahoma.*

Dr. Bob Ellis believed it was the right decision to move the Oklahoma Allergy Clinic to the Oklahoma Health Center even though many people still considered the campus to be in a less-than-desirable part of town. *Courtesy University of Oklahoma.*

For years the Oklahoma Allergy Clinic was located in the Pasteur Building on Northwest 10th Street across from St. Anthony Hospital. As with other practices, not all doctors in the clinic wanted to move. In part, the problem was one of perception—the Medical Center still was not considered to be located in the best part of town.

In 1977, the executive committee of the Oklahoma Health Sciences Foundation expressed concern about the deterioration of the area immediately west of OHC between Lincoln Boulevard and the Santa Fe Railroad, from Northeast 13th Street south. The Central Expressway, on the drawing board for years, was becoming a reality although the Oklahoma Highway Department had not yet decided exactly which route the expressway would traverse west of downtown. There was already $200 million of investment in OHC buildings, so foundation members were concerned about the less than desirable conditions in the area west of Lincoln.

In addition to the sad state of the neighborhood, the building of the Central Expressway, later named the Centennial Expressway to commemorate the Land Run of 1889, led to opposition in the community that feared neighborhoods would be divided by the highway. Ultimately, a "mitigation plan" addressed the concerns of the Harrison-Walnut Neighborhood Association and allowed the community to participate in the redevelopment of the area.

The acquisition of right-of-way for the Central Expressway provided the opportunity for OHC expansion. Stanton L. Young was a member of the State Highway Commission and helped expedite the sale of surplus right-of-way land to OHC, land that is now occupied by the Presbyterian Health Foundation Research Park. The Oklahoma Health Sciences Foundation purchased 45 parcels of land west of Lincoln Boulevard to protect and influence future land use which would relate to and complement the health

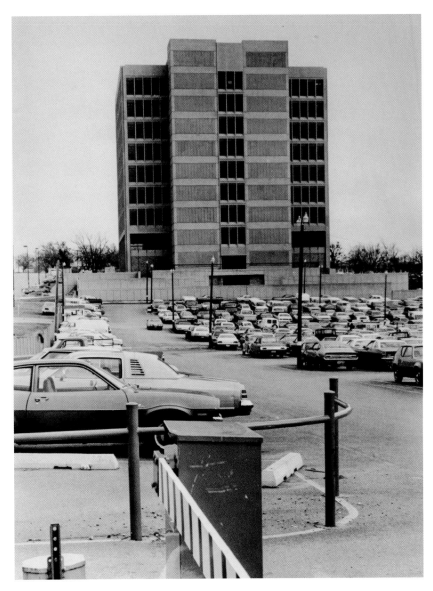

The 10-story Biomedical Sciences Building near Northeast 10th Street and Stonewall Avenue was completed in 1976. *Courtesy Oklahoma Publishing Company.*

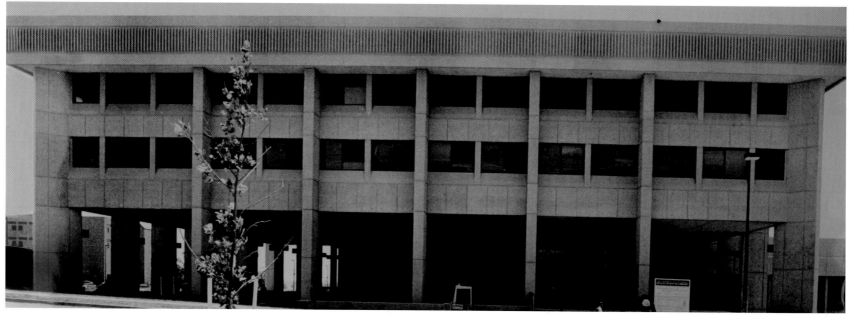

The new Robert M. Bird Library at the OU Health Sciences Center was dedicated in August, 1978. *Courtesy Oklahoma Publishing Company.*

campus. The mortgage was guaranteed by five civic leaders.

Although the decade of the 1970s was filled with funding and leadership difficulties, leaders never lost their dream for a comprehensive Oklahoma Health Center. Each time a problem arose, a solution was found.

A second surge of construction dramatically changed the OHC campus in 1980 and 1981. At one time in 1981, passersby could see construction cranes working on five different projects of more than $60 million, bringing total investment to more than $300 million. There was another $62 million in planned projects.

OU expanded the Dermatology Clinic and the steam and chilled water plant. The VA Medical Center began a $34 million addition. Down the street, Presbyterian Hospital built space in bays under the inpatient tower and extended the facility to the east for an ambulatory surgical center and a cancer center. OMRF expanded its north wing and OU renovated the old medical school building to house the Colleges of Public Health and Allied Health. The legislature appropriated more than $6 million to build a parking garage for the State Health Department. There was a clear-cut sign that officials were committed to a campus approach at the Oklahoma Health Center.

Hershel Lamirand arrived on the OHC campus in 1981 as Director of University Affairs to direct fund raising efforts at the OU Health Sciences Center. Lamirand had grown up in the

(Facing page) As new buildings went up in the medical center area in the late 1970s, and vacant lots or play space disappeared, students added a makeshift sign. *Courtesy Oklahoma Publishing Company.*

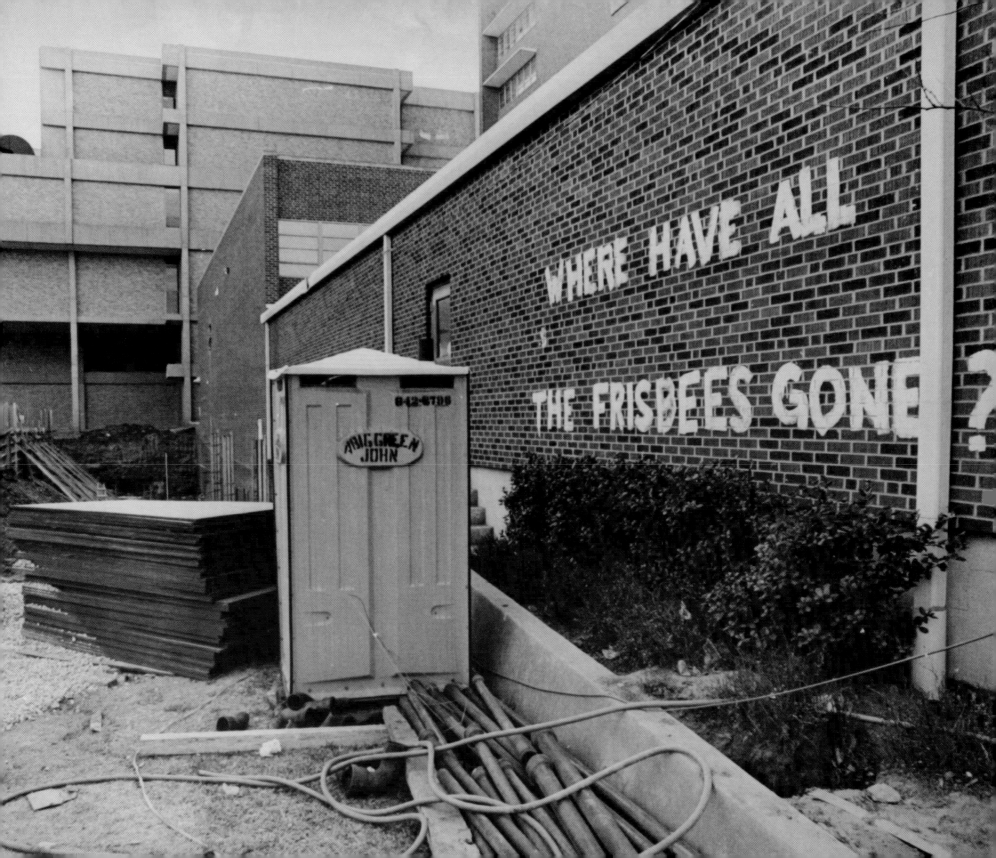

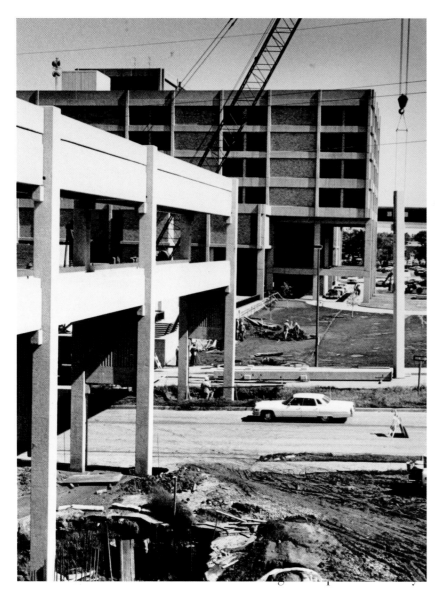

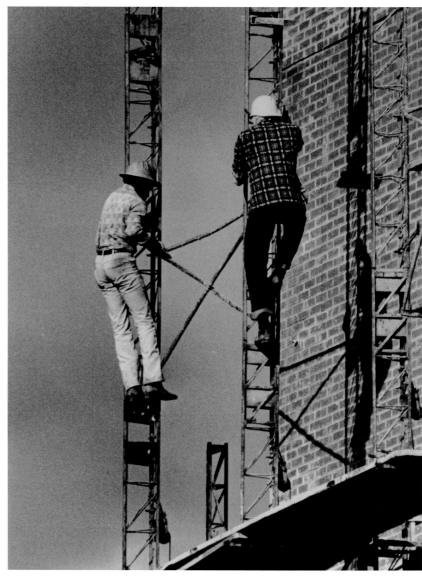

Growth of the mission of the Oklahoma Health Center was often measured by the amount of new construction. The sights of cranes and buildings going up excited supporters of the campus. *Courtesy Oklahoma Publishing Company.*

Workmen climb scaffolding during construction of the expansion at the Veterans Administration Medical Center in Oklahoma City in 1981. *Courtesy Oklahoma Publishing Company.*

Harrison-Walnut neighborhood, so working on the campus of OHC was like coming home. Lamirand began establishing relationships with the leadership of each of the campus institutions. Even though his primary job was to raise money for OU programs, he saw early in his career that the success or failure of the entire area depended upon the level of commitment to building a unified, world-class health care and research center.

OHC was reveling in an infusion of money from the state legislature because the state was in the middle of robust activity in the oil and gas business. Everyone seemed to have more money, the state unemployment rate was 3.7 percent, compared to more than eight percent nationwide, and the state was collecting more taxes than ever before.

Then, the economic boom went bust. Oklahoma City's Penn Square Bank, a symbol of the exuberance of drilling activity and oil hungry banks, failed. A sustained drop in energy prices caused petroleum and contract drilling companies to go bankrupt and the banking industry was severely injured. There were dire consequences for state government. Each reduction of $1 a barrel in the price of crude oil meant a $10 million drop in tax collections and another $143 million in pre-tax income for state producers.

When former Governor Henry Bellmon took the reins of the Department of Human Services (DHS), a new name for the Department of Public Welfare, on January 1, 1983, sales tax revenues were 25 percent below projections. A hiring freeze went into effect at DHS hospitals in the Oklahoma Health Center. Dr. Donald Halverstadt, administrator of University Hospital, was charged with cutting 400 staff positions.

In May, 1983, Robert Fulton replaced Bellmon and inherited the financial woes of the hospitals. Not only were revenues down,

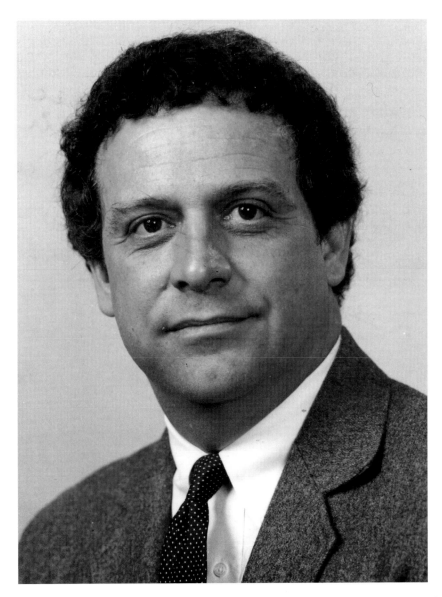

Hershel Lamirand came to the Oklahoma Health Center campus as Director of University Affairs at the OU Health Sciences Center in 1981. *Courtesy Oklahoma Publishing Company.*

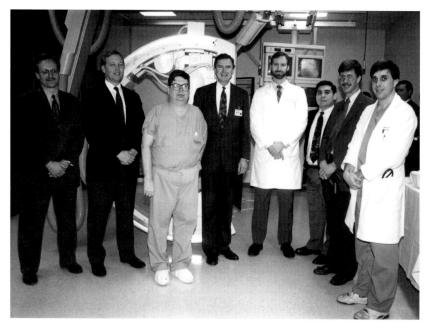

Presbyterian Hospital held a ribbon-cutting ceremony following the installation of a state-of-the-art Cardiac Catherization Laboratory. Left to right, Dr. Dwayne Schmidt, Dr. John Harvey, Dr. Thomas Russell, Presbyterian CEO David Dunlap, Dr. Angelo Ferraro, Dr. William Collazo, Dr. Alan Puls, and Dr. Thomas McGarry. *Courtesy Oklahoma Publishing Company.*

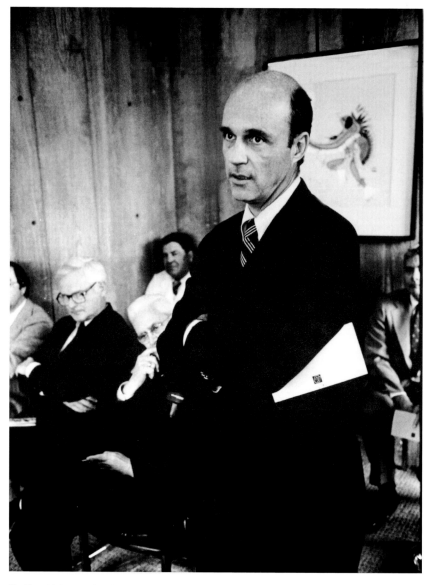

Dr. Don Halverstadt addresses a group attending the dedication of a new wing at the Dermatology Building on the OUHSC campus in 1981. Seate left are Dr. Clayton Rich and Lloyd Rader. *Courtesy Oklahoma Publishing Company.*

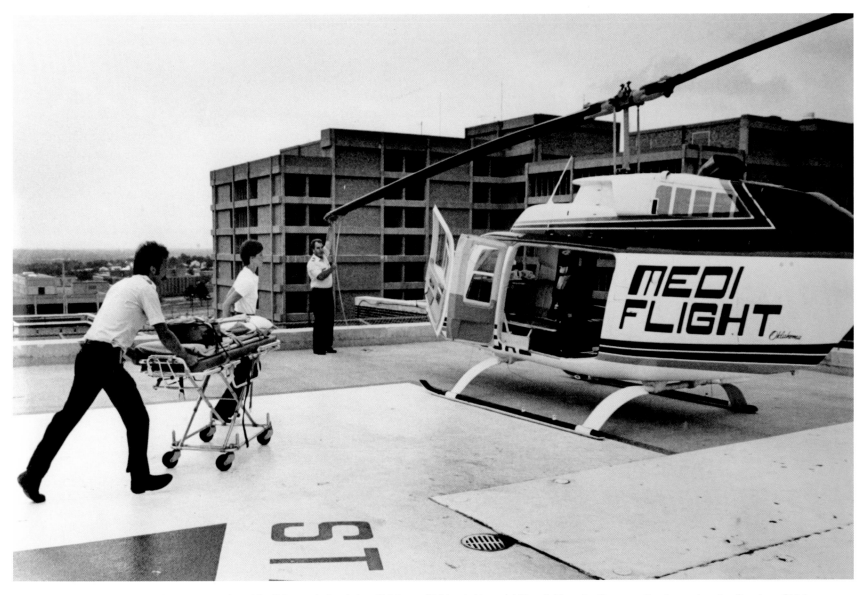

Medi Flight air ambulance attendants prepare for a lift-off from a helipad atop Oklahoma Children's Memorial Hospital in 1984. The operation began in 1980. *Courtesy Oklahoma Publishing Company.*

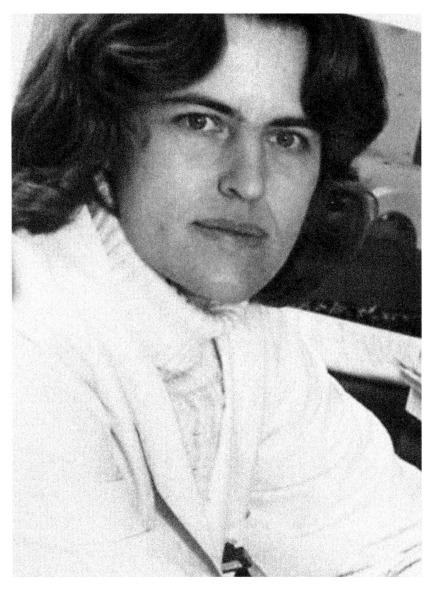

NASA selected Oklahoma Medical Research Foundation researcher, Dr. Shannon Lucid, as one of the world's first female astronauts. *Courtesy Oklahoma Medical Research Foundation.*

the average cost per patient was up. Somehow, DHS weathered the funding storm and quality hospital care continued.

The year 1983 saw improvements in the OHC and the surrounding neighborhood. Cars began parking in the new garage at the State Health Department. Construction began on the long-awaited Central Expressway. In early September, the VA Medical Center celebrated its new addition west of the original building and OMRF held open house at its new cardiovascular research building.

In early October, Presbyterian Hospital kicked off festivities to open the Bob Hope Eye Surgery Center. The 80-year-old entertainer addressed an enthusiastic crowd of potential donors at the Skirvin Plaza Hotel. In November, the $7.5 million, 70,000 square foot home of the OU College of Pharmacy was officially opened. The major private donation came from Henry and Ida Mosier, an Edmond couple for whom the building was named. Mr. Mosier was a 1912 graduate of the college.

Children's Medical Research, Inc., now Children's Medical Research Institute (CMRI), began operation on the OHC campus in 1983. CMRI is the only organization in Oklahoma whose only focus is the advancement of pediatric research and education. The organization was born three years earlier during a Christmas Party conversation between Dr. Owen Rennert, a pediatrician and interim chief of staff at the Oklahoma Teaching Hospitals, and Jean Gumerson. Dr. Rennert believed the success of the Department of Pediatrics at the hospitals would be helped by the formation of a foundation to assist in funding.

Gumerson facilitated a meeting between First Lady Donna Nigh, who was interested in children's programs, and civic leaders James Paul Linn, John Kilpatrick, and Robert Fulton, director of the Department of Human Services. A non-profit foundation

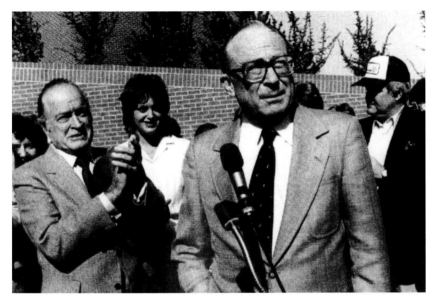

Comedian Bob Hope, left, and publisher Edward L. Gaylord help dedicate the Bob Hope Eye Surgery Center at Presbyterian Hospital in 1983. *Courtesy Oklahoma Publishing Company.*

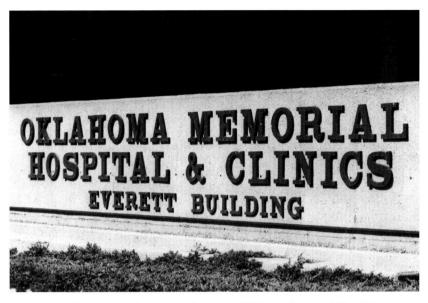

In 1985, the old University Hospital was known as Oklahoma Memorial Hospital. *Courtesy Oklahoma Publishing Company.*

was created which began to provide lay leadership to support the Children's Hospital and the Department of Pediatrics. Gumerson served as the early chair of CMRI's board whose goal was to raise sufficient funds to endow five chairs in pediatric research in the OU College of Medicine.

In early 1984, Governor George Nigh and the Oklahoma legislature considered further spending cuts, in light of reduced state tax collections. An audit of the Oklahoma Teaching Hospitals called for restructuring the management of the hospitals. Oklahoma Memorial Hospital, a new name for University Hospital, had completed three additional floors and operated 361 beds. The legislature passed three new tax measures to increase state

revenues. Even with new revenues, it was a time of belt-tightening and deferral of new programs for the tenants of the OHC that depended upon state appropriations.

With the dismal financial news, there was no doubt that the Oklahoma Health Center was making an impact upon Oklahoma. By 1984, the Center had grown to ten institutions, seven colleges, 35 buildings, and more than 2,500 students on 200 acres. It had been a 20-year running start to develop and expand health education and manpower for the state and broaden medical research programs and patient care. The investment in OHC had surpassed $350 million and the cost of operating all the institutions on the campus exceeded a half billion dollars annually.

Chapter Four

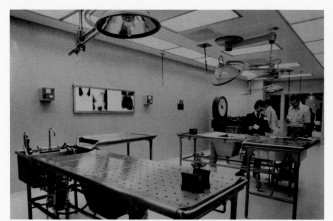 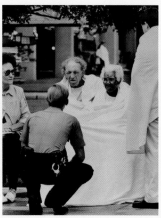 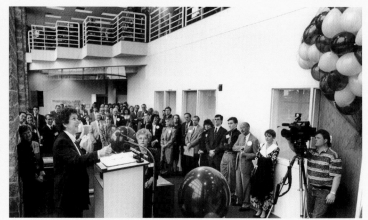

Changing Times

The first two decades of growth on the OHC campus was paying dividends. Health care workers were graduating in record numbers. Student numbers in the OU medical, nursing, dentistry, and pharmacy colleges continued to increase. Not only were admissions up, applications for the limited number of spots in the professional schools also increased.

From 1982 to 1984, research grants increased in the OU College of Public Health from $300,000 to $1.5 million. Faculty was added and laboratory equipment was upgraded to make space for competing for federal grants in environmental health. Other components of the OU Health Sciences Center reported similar increases in research grants.

At the Oklahoma Medical Research Foundation, Executive Director Dr. Bill Thurman developed and implemented an incremental 10-, 15-, and 20-year plan, charting where OMRF was going and what it would need to get there. Across the campus at the Dean McGee Eye Institute, Dr. Tom Acers drafted a 10-year expansion program to carry the institute into the next decade. Its namesake, Dean McGee, was overjoyed at the early success of the institute. McGee said, "It has met and exceeded my expectations of developing a really first class eye institute to serve the middle part of the country."

The Oklahoma City Clinic was serving the most patients ever, and the VA Medical Center used a van to carry doctors to outlying state homes and communities to assess veterans who might need long term care. Dr. Joan Leavitt, State Commissioner of Health, championed the state's continuing effort to decentralize the public health network out in the counties.

Soaring health care costs caused federal and state governments and hospitals to reconsider their relationships in the 1980s. By 1984, Congress feared the Social Security program, including Medicare, was going broke and mandated sweeping changes in the way hospitals were paid. Rather than paying for Medicaid and Medicare patients' actual treatment costs, the government began reimbursing hospitals based upon the patient's illness, not on the

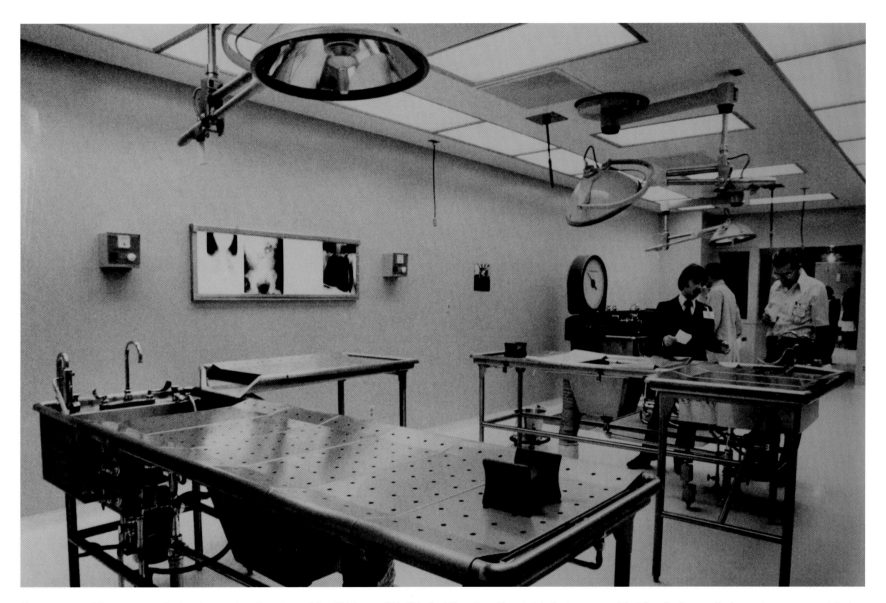

New autopsy tables were installed at the new headquarters of the Oklahoma Chief Medical Examiner. The state's first permanent building for the medical examiner was completed in 1978 at Northeast 8th Street and Stonewall Avenue. *Courtesy Oklahoma Publishing Company.*

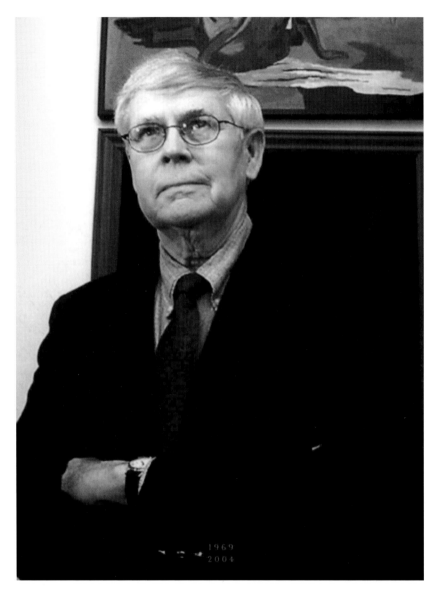

Dr. Mark Allen Everett was the son of the medical school dean, Dr. Mark Everett. Both played integral roles in the development of the Oklahoma Health Center. *Courtesy Oklahoma Publishing Company.*

length of time he or she stays in the hospital or how many tests or treatments were given. Illnesses were classified into 467 diagnosis-related groups (DRGs) and hospitals were reimbursed on the average cost of treating patients with these medical programs which differed in nine regions of the country.

The Medicare prospective pricing system caused hospital officials to look for ways to cut costs. The problems were faced head-on by the board of Oklahoma City's Presbyterian Hospital where the number of patients had declined. In addition, trustees were servicing a large debt left over from building the new hospital on the OHC campus. Presbyterian had the highest nurse-to-patient ratio among private hospitals in the Oklahoma City area. If that high level of care was to continue, Stanton L. Young said, there had to be a new source of revenue.

Dennis McGrath, chief financial officer of Presbyterian Hospital, told trustees that the hospital could not compete with the other major hospitals in town on the basis of costs. Baptist and Saint Anthony hospitals had little debt.

To cut the cost of health care, large, health care delivery systems were invented. Health Corporation of America (HCA) was the largest health care system in the world and growing very fast. HCA saw preferred provider organizations (PPOs) as a way to regain market share which had steadily eroded through competition. HCA had acquired some flagship hospitals and wanted to increase its presence in larger markets such as Oklahoma City.

Presbyterian Hospital board chairman Young invited HCA officials to take a look at the Oklahoma City facility that was spending $6 million a year on debt service alone. With the original construction costs and other capital expenditures, the debt was approximately $58 million. It was the beginning of a landmark hospital sale that has had an unbelievable positive impact upon the economy of Oklahoma City and the State of Oklahoma.

It was a seller's market. In October, 1984, HCA and Presbyterian Hospital signed a letter of intent to sell the hospital. After months of negotiations, HCA offered to pay $125 million for the facility. Dr. Michael Anderson, Westminster Presbyterian Church pastor and a Presbyterian Hospital trustee since 1977, remembered the joy the HCA bid gave trustees. He said, "We saw the opportunity of getting out of the business of running a hospital and getting back into a different non-profit mission with net proceeds of $64 million."

Presbyterian Hospital President Harry Neer told reporters that the intended sale marked a major development in hospital care in Oklahoma. HCA owned 400 hospitals in 44 states, but most facilities were only half the size of Presbyterian. In Oklahoma, HCA owned Edmond Memorial Hospital and Wagoner Community Hospital and operated St. Mary's Hospital in Enid. After approval of the Indian Nations Presbytery of the Presbyterian Church and the Oklahoma Health Planning Commission, the sale of Presbyterian Hospital was complete in July, 1985.

Before the sale of the hospital was complete, Dr. Anderson chaired a long-range planning committee and developed a plan for the Presbyterian Health Foundation (PHF) to wisely invest and spend the $64 million available after paying the hospital's debt. It was decided at the foundation's first meeting the proceeds realized from the sale of the hospital would be used to improve the quality of medical education and research in Oklahoma. None of the trustees could foresee that PHF would become the largest donor to the programs of the University of Oklahoma and would cast a vision for private sector research impacting Oklahoma for generations.

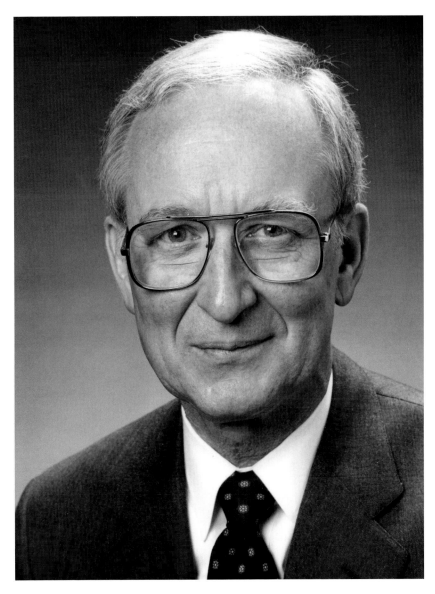

Ed Miller, president of Founders National Bank in Oklahoma City, was the first chairman of the Presbyterian Health Foundation board of directors. *Courtesy Oklahoma Publishing Company.*

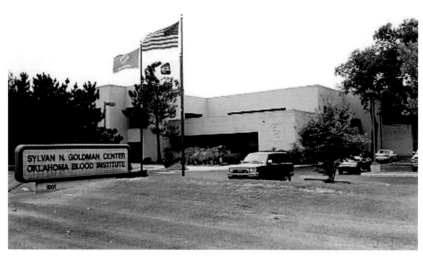

The home of the Oklahoma Blood Institute on the Oklahoma Health Center campus. *Courtesy Oklahoma Blood Institute.*

After the sale of Presbyterian Hospital to HCA, the Oklahoma Health Center enjoyed a period of relative quiet for the remainder of the 1980s. Most of the institutions on campus were consolidating their gains and learning to live with expanded facilities. Dean McGee said, "After a spurt of growth, all organizations need a period during which they can digest the expansion they have achieved and improve their operations at a new level."

One of the additions to the OHC campus area in 1984 was the Ronald McDonald House at 1301 Northeast 14th Street. The House offers a caring retreat to families of children undergoing treatment at nearby Children's Hospital. A volunteer board of directors guides Ronald McDonald House Charities of Oklahoma City and raises money to finance and operate the House and fund grant and scholarship programs.

Officials at the OU Health Sciences Center realized future growth revolved around research programs. In three years, from 1982 to 1985, external funding for research tripled. Twenty-two faculty members received research funds of more than $100,000 through competitive projects.

The growth of research had been at the top of Dr. Clayton Rich's list of priorities when he became provost of the OUHSC in 1980. Rich credited faculty efforts for the remarkable surge in research activity which topped $15 million in grants and contracts in 1985.

The emphasis on research at OUHSC drew favorable comment from business and civic leaders in Oklahoma City and around the state. They recognized the quality of research being conducted at the Health Sciences Center would have a positive impact on the economic development of the region. Dr. Rich and community leaders looked forward to a day when high-technology industries—and the jobs that come with them—would be attracted to medical centers involved in research development and marketing of new products and techniques.

The community's interest in research programs at OHC was frequently documented by news coverage. An article in *The Daily Oklahoman* on March 14, 1986, announced $2 million in endowment gifts to support programs in eye care and surgery. A $1 million gift from Dorothy Miller went to the Department of Surgery and a $1 million gift from Edward L. Gaylord, president of the Oklahoma Publishing Company, established the Gaylord Chair of Ophthalmology to support teaching programs at the OU College of Ophthalmology and the Dean A. McGee Eye Institute.

One of the few blips on the sea of tranquility at the Oklahoma Health Center came in the State of the State message of Oklahoma Governor Henry Bellmon in January, 1987. Bellmon, faced with a

$350 million shortfall of tax revenues, was looking for places to cut state appropriations, and he focused on the OU College of Dentistry.

Bellmon, in his second term as governor, proposed that the College of Dentistry be closed. He reasoned that it was costing the state $5 million annually. He said, "The dental school wasn't being picked on—it just looked to us as a way to save the taxpayers a significant amount of money."

The most shocked person in the state was College of Dentistry Dean Bill Brown. He had spent 18 years of his life planning, designing, building, and operating the dental school. By 1985, the dental school had cut back substantially on its enrollment to 50 new students each year versus 72 students in previous years, a mandate from the Department of Health, Education, and Welfare as a condition of taking federal money to construct the building. The first class graduated in 1976.

Dean Brown and his staff had no contact with the governor. Bellmon would talk only with OU President Frank Horton about the idea of closing the dental school. However, Brown produced single-page fact sheets and asked staff, students, and patients to write letters to their legislators. State Representatives Carolyn Thompson and Vicki White, who was married to a dental school graduate, began developing a plan in the legislature to oppose Bellmon's move to close the dental school. House Speaker Jim Barker announced his support to keep the school open even as rumors spread that the dental school was of poor quality and unnecessary to supply Oklahoma with well-trained dentists.

A report generated by OU showed that there was no advantage in closing the dental school. In fact, there were several disadvantages. Oklahoma was 20 percent below the national average in dentist-patient ratio, and there was no reasonable belief the shortage of dentists would be filled by dentists coming from other states. Also, if the dental school was closed, it would force the elimination of 37,000 dental clinic visits per year of people who could pay only part or none of the cost of their care. The College of Dentistry also provided a valuable service of continuing education for practicing dentists in the state.

The legislature won the battle over Governor Bellmon. During the final days of the legislative session, legislative leaders effectively killed any plan to close the dental school. As the state's population increased, the need for dentists and specialists in oral and maxilla-facial surgery, orthodontics, and periodontics increased. The near-closing of the school was emotionally draining but fortified the school stronger and expanded its private donor base.

The institution occupying the largest single space on the Oklahoma Health Center campus is the Oklahoma School of Science and Mathematics (OSSM). The creation of the school came after a five-year battle resulting with the opening of classes in 1990 on the 32-acre campus on the west side of Lincoln Boulevard, an area once the site of a deteriorating, crime-ridden neighborhood.

The idea was to establish a residential school to train some of the state's brightest high school students. The governor's education coordinator, Dr. Carolyn Smith, was a major force in keeping the issue alive as a monumental battle developed over the location of OSSM.

The bill to establish a residential public school for advanced science and mathematics high school students was authored by Representative Penny Williams and Senate President Pro Tempore Rodger Randle, both of Tulsa. OSSM was authorized by the legislature in 1983 with the support of Governor George Nigh after a group of lawmakers visited the North Carolina School of Science and Mathematics in Durham, North Carolina.

In 1986, Governor Nigh appointed 25 educators, business leaders, and legislators to the newly created Board of Trustees for OSSM with Madill attorney Dan Little as the first chairman of the board. When it looked as if OSSM might become a reality, several communities applied for the school. Within a short time, the "short list" of cities where OSSM might be located was Oklahoma City, Edmond, Stillwater, and Norman. OU Department of Medicine's Dr. Patrick McKee was a major representative on the board from OHC and promoted the establishment of OSSM to show gifted students Oklahoma was committed to keeping its brightest and best.

The decision of where to locate OSSM was politically charged. It was rumored incoming Governor Bellmon promised the school would be built on a 400-acre site near the Oklahoma State University campus in Stillwater. Two locations were touted in Oklahoma City: the former campus of Midwest Christian College at Northeast 63rd Street and Kelly Avenue and 32 acres between Lincoln Boulevard and the Centennial Expressway. Battle lines formed.

At about the same time, Hershel Lamirand, Bill Pirtle, and Stanton L. Young visited Dean McGee in his elaborate office atop the Kerr-McGee Building in downtown Oklahoma City. McGee was concerned that the Oklahoma Health Center Foundation had "gone to sleep." The original purposes of the Health Center had been accomplished and the foundation was resting on its laurels. Lamirand, whose primary job was to raise money for the OU Health Sciences Center, accepted the invitation of McGee and Young to rebuild the foundation board. The change ignited a rebirth of the efforts of the foundation—and locating OSSM was the OHC battle cry.

Lamirand began using his contacts in Leadership Oklahoma City to build a template for the foundation that would allow the chief executive officers of the 14 institutions that made up the Oklahoma Health Center to rub elbows on a regular basis with civic, government, and business leaders. Two thirds of the new foundation board members were younger leaders who wanted to make a difference. Lamirand remembered, "All at once, we had a forum—a place where city and state government, the business community, and university leaders could sit down and promote a cause for the common good. The first cause was OSSM."

The heart of the plan was to locate OSSM on the OHC campus surrounded by Ebenezer Baptist Church and Lincoln Elementary School, the two structures remaining on the 32 acres west of Lincoln Boulevard. Oklahoma City's plan was presented to the OSSM Board of Trustees by Dr. Ann Ackerman of Oklahoma City Community College and in Class 5 of Leadership Oklahoma City.

Norman and Edmond were eliminated from the selection process, and only Oklahoma City and Stillwater vied for the school. In December, 1987, three independent consultants recommended Oklahoma City as the best location. But Senator Bernice Shedrick of Stillwater lobbied heavily for the site near the OSU campus. There was political tension in the air as board members were split evenly, 9-9. There was an unbreakable impasse and the board adjourned without a decision.

The following month, in January, 1988, trustees voted 10-9 to locate OSSM on the Oklahoma Health Center campus. Trustee and Senator Penny Williams cast the deciding vote. "It was a courageous vote," remembered Lamirand. "Everyone assumed she would vote in favor of Stillwater because of her long friendship with Senator Shedrick. However, she voted for Oklahoma City because it was the right thing to do."

With the decision to build OSSM in Oklahoma City, civic

leaders pledged to raise $1.5 million in private funds to renovate the closed Lincoln Elementary School. The city council of Oklahoma City, led by City Councilman Pete White, promised to pay $2 million needed for campus infrastructure. Leaders also expressed their willingness to work with the legislature to secure an additional $10 million to complete the campus.

The Daily Oklahoman editorially applauded the selection of Oklahoma City for OSSM, one of only four specialized schools of its kind in the nation. The editorial said, "One of the major selling points for the Oklahoma City site was the promised access for the students to the medical center." On the other hand, the *Tulsa World* labeled the new school a "big, tax-gobbling turkey." Ultimately, the state legislature funded construction projects to ready the school for occupancy.

Edna Manning, the former school superintendent in Shawnee, was chosen to head OSSM and its 52 students in September, 1990. It had taken seven years to secure a location and funding for the innovative school. The success of the board in uniting business, university, and government leaders in the effort to win OSSM for the Oklahoma Health Center campus would be replicated many times in the following decade.

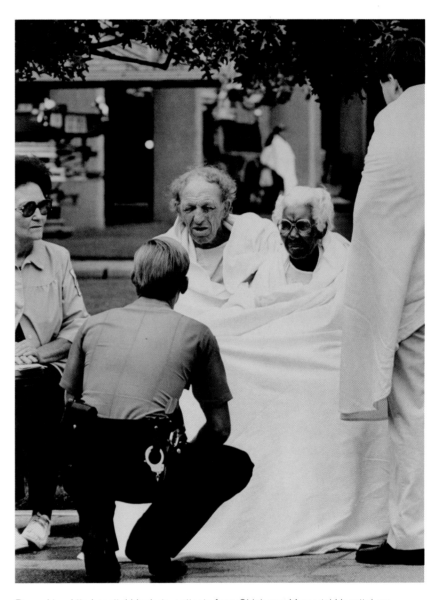

Draped in white hospital blankets, patients from Oklahoma Memorial Hospital are comforted by a police officer until they get the all clear to return following a fire in October, 1988. More than 800 patients and staff were forced to leave because of the basement blaze. *Courtesy Oklahoma Publishing Company.*

The unique architecture of the interior of the Oklahoma School of Science and Mathematics creates an atmosphere conducive to learning. *Courtesy Oklahoma Publishing Company.*

Bright Students, Bright Future

Only one of a handful of high schools of its kind in the nation, the Oklahoma School of Science and Mathematics flourishes as a unique learning institution for Oklahoma students. Created through legislative action and signed into law by Governor George Nigh in 1983, the residential public high school was founded on the principle of providing academically advanced junior and senior students with college-level courses in science and math, as well as fostering educational development in other subjects.

Situated on a 32-acre campus near the Oklahoma Health Center in Oklahoma City, OSSM, classified as a state agency, serves all schools and students through research, summer teacher training and outreach activities.

Attorney Dan Little of Madill is the first and only chairman of the OSSM Board of Trustees. Mr. Little has been influential in his support for OSSM over the years and the school's residential dormitory is named in his honor.

Dr. Earl Mitchell, retired professor from Oklahoma State University, and currently a member of the OSSM Board of Trustees, along with Senator Penny Williams, of Tulsa, were two of the driving forces behind the creation of OSSM. Senator Bernice Shedrick, of Stillwater, was also one of OSSM's staunchest supporters in the senate during the years the school was struggling for its existence in the state legislature. The school's library is named in honor of Senator Shedrick. All three continue to champion OSSM.

Although the history of the school is grand, the wonderfully gifted students are the heart of OSSM. Since its inception, graduates have come from all 77 counties throughout Oklahoma. It was not easy for early students. The Class of 1990-1991 attended classes at the Oklahoma Health Center, as well as the

University of Oklahoma, and lived in dormitories on OU's Norman campus until the restoration of Lincoln School was completed in December of 1991. Much of the school's interior construction was left exposed, with the architect's conceptions of early Greek and Roman designs added. The original hardwood maple floors in classrooms and brick walls of the former boiler room remain intact.

Students continued to live in temporary quarters and commuted from Norman to Oklahoma City until the Dan Little Residence Hall opened in 1998. The next year, the gymnasium was constructed, followed by The Samson Science and Discovery Center and the Senator Bernice Shedrick Library.

The graduates of OSSM have already left their indelible marks on Oklahoma. Of the 1,024 OSSM graduates since the first class, 297 former students are engineers and 58 are medical doctors, plus 100 more alumni in each of these fields are currently completing their studies. Eighty-five percent of these graduates have careers in science, math, engineering and technology. More than half now work or live in the state, and nine graduates have begun their own businesses in Oklahoma.

Yet, behind these bright minds are exceptional faculty members. OSSM boasts 40 faculty and staff from all over the world, including 23 professors with doctorates and 12 with master's degrees, many of whom have taught at prestigious universities before joining the school. Curriculum is tailored to provide a scholastic program of excellence in the sciences and mathematics, as well as exemplary instructional courses in humanities, the arts and physical education. Interestingly, two of the school's graduates are now faculty members.

The school's residency program is designed to encourage an atmosphere of informal interaction among peers and foster each student's highest potential. The availability of laboratories, along with evening and weekend programs of interest, challenge students and stimulate studies. About 40 percent of seniors now complete mentorships with researchers and scientists from the Oklahoma Health Center, local universities and private firms.

The success of OSSM depends on a unique partnership of public and private support. This is accomplished through the OSSM Foundation, which augments the finances of the school through charitable donations, including a faculty endowment. The ultimate goal for OSSM is to establish an enrollment of 300 students, doubling its current size. Private funds have already been raised to expand the existing dormitory; however, additional funding is needed from the state legislature to ensure the school's future and keep the dream alive for Oklahoma's best and brightest students.

Dr. Edna Manning,
President
Oklahoma School of Science and Mathematics

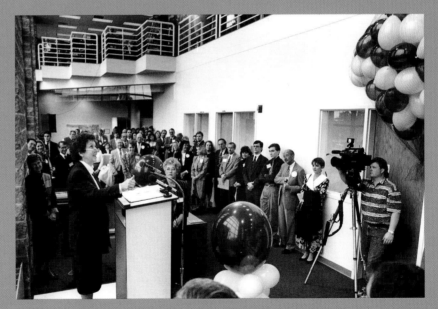

Dr. Edna Manning, president of the Oklahoma School of Science and Mathematics, speaks at the school's dedication ceremony in 1992. *Courtesy Oklahoma Publishing Company.*

Chapter Five

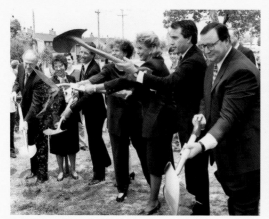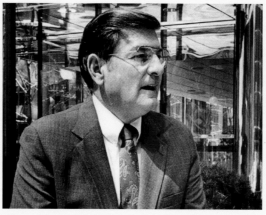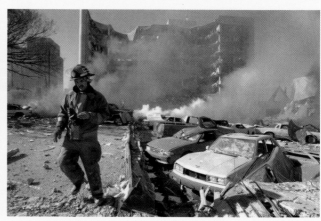

The Giant Awakens

Fresh from winning the monumental battle
to locate the Oklahoma School of Science and
Mathematics in Oklahoma City, the Oklahoma
Health Center Foundation began to flex its muscles
to promote further development of the
OHC campus.

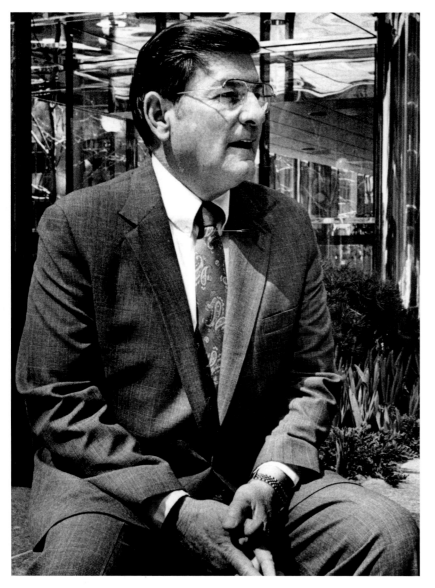

William "Bill" Pirtle, senior vice president of Oklahoma Natural Gas Company, became president of the Oklahoma Health Center Foundation board and sparked new interest in promoting the campus and its occupants. *Courtesy Oklahoma Publishing Company.*

*D*uring discussions of reviving the foundation's role in developing the campus, Dean McGee suggested that his dreams and the vision of other leaders be carried on by the next generation. Stanton L. Young and others suggested Oklahoma Natural Gas Company Senior Vice President William N. "Bill" Pirtle serve as president. Pirtle accepted the charge from stalwart leaders such as Edward L. Gaylord, Harvey Everest, and McGee.

Under Pirtle's direction, the foundation board began meeting regularly and redefined its role, and officially changed its name to the Oklahoma Health Center Foundation. The chief executive officers of the OHC member institutions met and began working together to solve common problems. Revised articles of incorporation required CEOs on the operations committee to appear for meetings personally, rather than send subordinates.

One of the first projects of the new foundation board was to market the Oklahoma Health Center. Volunteers from Kerr-McGee Corporation, the Oklahoma Publishing Company, and Jordan and Associates Advertising contributed their time to the effort. The board also worked to develop an overall plan for the campus.

In 1988, Dr. Clayton Rich, provost of the OU Health Sciences Center, authored a paper comparing the OUHSC to "world class medical centers"—institutions affiliated with Duke University, Harvard College, Johns Hopkins University, Stanford University, and the University of Washington.

Rich found that the size and quality of the OU teaching hospitals, the clinical and educational programs, and facilities of the various health professional colleges were adequate and compared favorably to top-tier medical centers in the nation. The survey found that the only critical difference between OUHSC and other top quality medical centers was the research output by medical

Rebirth of the Oklahoma Health Center Foundation

In the late 1980s, the Oklahoma Health Center Foundation board of trustees was recreated. Dean McGee was the only member of the original Oklahoma Health Sciences Foundation board in 1966.

Members in 1990 included:

William N. Pirtle, President
Dr. Virginia Hendrick, Vice President
Stanton L. Young, Vice President
Hershel Lamirand, Secretary
Stanley A. Lybarger, Treasurer
Robert C. Hardy, Assistant Secretary
Dr. Ann Ackerman
Robert H. Alexander, Jr.
William M. Bell
Dr. John Bozalis
Bill Cameron
Richard H. Clements
Douglas R. Cummings
Richard D. Harrison

Clyde Ingle
Lou Kerr
Jill King
Stephen Lynn
Dean McGee
Ed Miller
Dr. Don O'Donoghue
Russell Perry
David Rainbolt
Carol Wilkinson
Dr. G. Rainey Williams
Lee Young
Ron Yordi

The chief executive officers of the Oklahoma Health Center institutions were then considered ex-officio members of the executive committee of the OHC Foundation. They were:

Thomas E. Acers—Dean A. McGee Eye Institute
David Dunlap—HCA Presbyterian Hospital
Steven J. Gentling—Veterans Administration Hospital
Dr. J. Frank James—Oklahoma Department of Mental Health
Dr. Andy Lasser—Oklahoma Medical Center
Dr. Joan K. Leavitt—Oklahoma Department of Health

Keith Montgomery—Oklahoma Allergy Clinic
Dr. Willard B. Moran—Oklahoma City Clinic
Dr. Clayton Rich—OU Health Sciences Center
Dr. William G. Thurman—Oklahoma Medical Research Foundation
Phil Watson—Oklahoma Department of Human Services

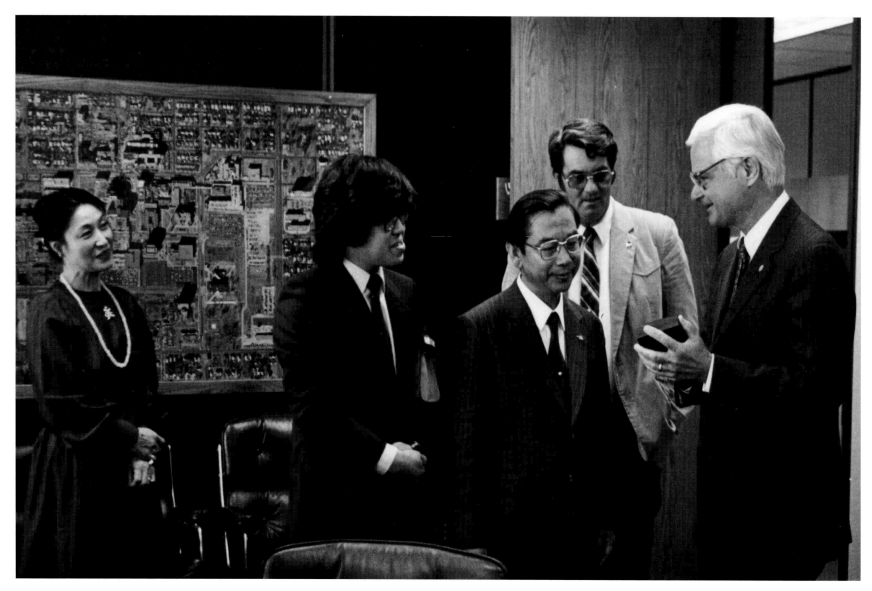

Provost Clayton Rich, right, welcomes Japanese visitors to the OUHSC campus. *Courtesy Robert M. Bird Health Sciences Library.*

school faculty. Rich concluded that the only thing needed to make the OU medical center world class was a sharp increase in the amount and quality of research in the College of Medicine.

In order to accomplish a significant increase in research, the provost suggested:

1. Raising state funding to the national average;
2. Establishing a special fund of $600,000 per year to recruit top quality scientists to the College of Medicine;
3. Increasing private support, particularly from Oklahoma foundations;
4. Building a new research building with 117,000 net square feet of laboratory space; and
5. Maintaining university and statewide policies that promote research development.

Dr. Rich explained the purpose of releasing his paper at that time. He said, "Top quality was really the goal I was aiming for. The quality of people you recruit throughout the faculty is dependent on how faculty generally look at your school. A school which is full of really bright, interesting people who are doing interesting, worthwhile things is attractive to faculty."

At the time Dr. Rich wrote his World Class Medical Center paper, OU had achieved recruiting good scientists in basic sciences and nearly all laboratory space was occupied. The biomedical sciences building was a nice research building, but it was too small for the development of research in a modern medical school.

OUHSC officials began working with federal and state agencies, including a second round of HERO bonds, to raise sufficient monies for capital projects. The state budget had never fully recovered

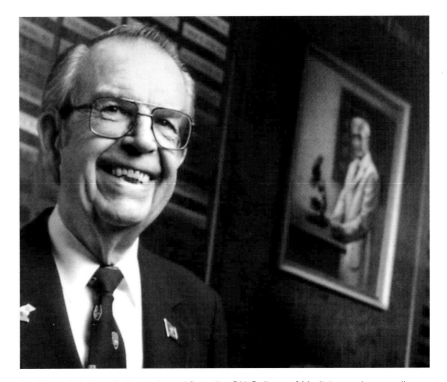

Dr. Edward N. Brandt, Jr., graduated from the OU College of Medicine and was well qualified to become dean in 1989. When Brandt died in 2007, OUHSC Provost Dr. Joseph Ferretti called him "the most highly recognized and most important contributor to medicine and public health of any individual ever associated with the University of Oklahoma." *Courtesy University of Oklahoma.*

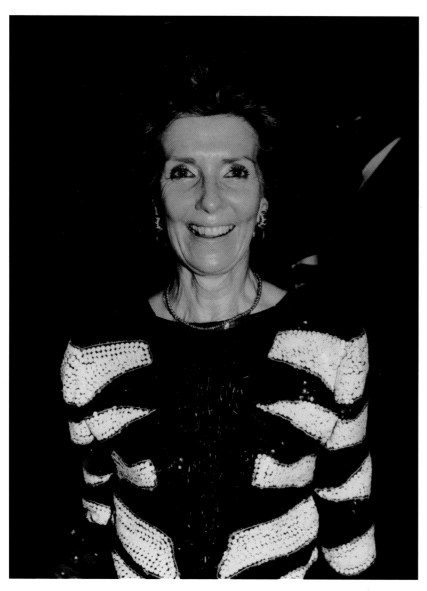

Jean Gumerson was a veteran not-for-profit administrator when she became president of the Presbyterian Health Foundation. *Courtesy Oklahoma Publishing Company.*

from the oil bust of the middle 1980s, and the operational budget was not adequate. Even with budgetary problems, official began to look for ways to engage OUHSC in heavy biomedical research.

Dr. Edward N. Brandt, Jr., replaced Dr. Donald G. Kassebaum as Dean of the OU College of Medicine in 1989. Brandt, a graduate of the OU medical school in 1960, was well qualified for the position. He served as Assistant United States Secretary of Health, acting Surgeon General of the United States, vice chancellor of the University of Texas Medical Center, and president of the University of Baltimore.

Brandt had worked at the OUHSC as associate dean of the medical school in the 1960s and was disappointed at the lack of state government's excitement over the importance of medical education and research. When he returned in 1989, he saw Governor Bellmon and state leaders taking a fresh look at higher education. Brandt believed his major job at the medical school was to improve morale, encourage the faculty to believe in themselves, and recognize they could change things. He envisioned the Oklahoma Health Center as becoming a more potent economic force.

Brandt also believed in the OUHSC goal of becoming a world class medical center. He pushed programs that blended research with patient care. Brandt said, "If we have faculty who basically do nothing but research or whose only interest is research, and do not pay any attention to education, that will be bad." Brandt warned of developing separate faculty for research, teaching, and patient care.

In 1989, Ed Miller, president of the Presbyterian Health Foundation, died. Dr. Michael Anderson and other trustees of the foundation encouraged Jean Gumerson to make application to succeed Miller. Gumerson was well qualified and was hired. She was a director of the Children's Medical Research Foundation and had previously served as executive director of the Oklahoma Art Center and director of public relations for the C.R. Anthony Company.

By 1990, the Presbyterian Health Foundation had become a major donor for programs at the OU Health Sciences Center. In June, 1990, PHF granted $818,602 to OUHSC for medical research. Dr. O. Ray Kling, interim vice provost for research, announced the receipt of the grant which he said would fund 16 projects. The money from PHF allowed young researchers at OUHSC to develop nationally competitive research programs.

In addition to the large grant, PHF also provided funds for the purchase of equipment and establishment of the medical scholars program that gave students the opportunity to do research during the summer.

Success breeds success. As PHF money became available to assist programs at OUHSC, other supporters of OU and medical research came forward. An example in 1991 was PHF adding $150,000 to a $400,000 gift from the Ungerman Trust of Tulsa to establish an endowed chair in cross-cultural psychiatric care at OUHSC. The $500,000 was then matched by the Oklahoma State Regents for Higher Education to provide $1 million for the endowed chair which was named for Dr. Arnold H. Ungerman, a 1934 OU College of Medicine graduate, who practiced as a psychiatrist on the Navajo Indian Reservation and in Tulsa.

To inform the public of increased activity at the Oklahoma Health Center, television news anchor and former Miss America Jane Jayroe was hired in 1992 to prepare programs for the media and help recruit researchers, scientists, and teaching faculty to Oklahoma. In weekly programs aired on Oklahoma City and Tulsa television stations, research projects and medical programs were explained by guests. During one week, "Jane Jayroe's Medical Journal" featured a compelling story of a patient's struggle

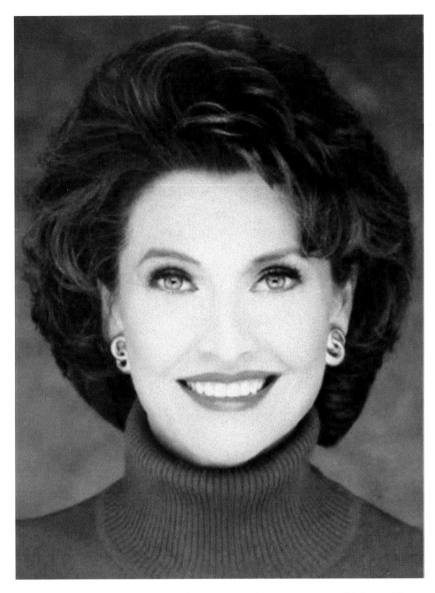

Former Miss America Jane Jayroe left her news anchor position at an Oklahoma City television station to become a spokesperson for the Oklahoma Health Center. *Courtesy Oklahoma Heritage Association.*

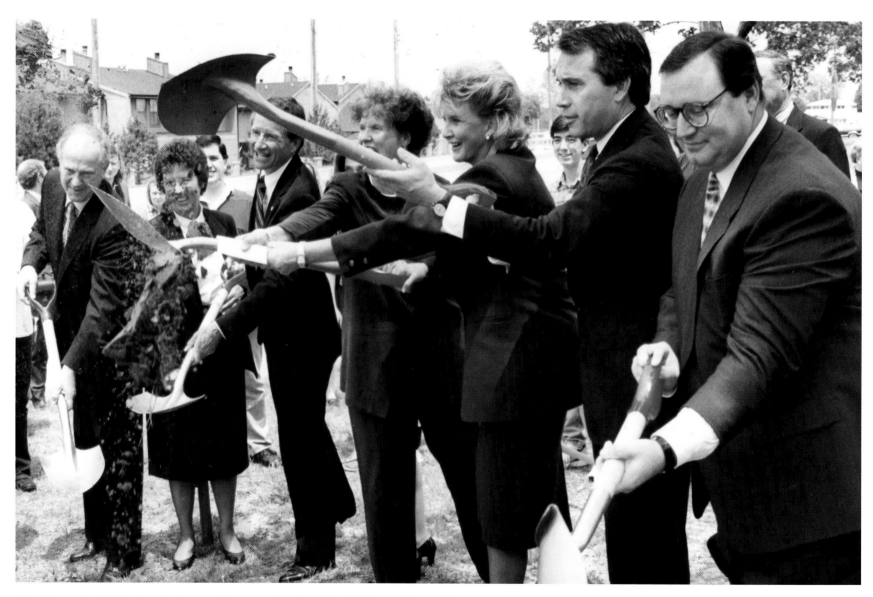

Education and political leaders break ground for a new dormitory at the Oklahoma School of Science and Mathematics in 1994. Left to right, Richard Bell, Dr. Edna Manning, Dan Little, Senator Penny Williams, Senator Bernice Shedrick, Governor David Walters, and House Speaker Glen Johnson. *Courtesy Oklahoma Publishing Company.*

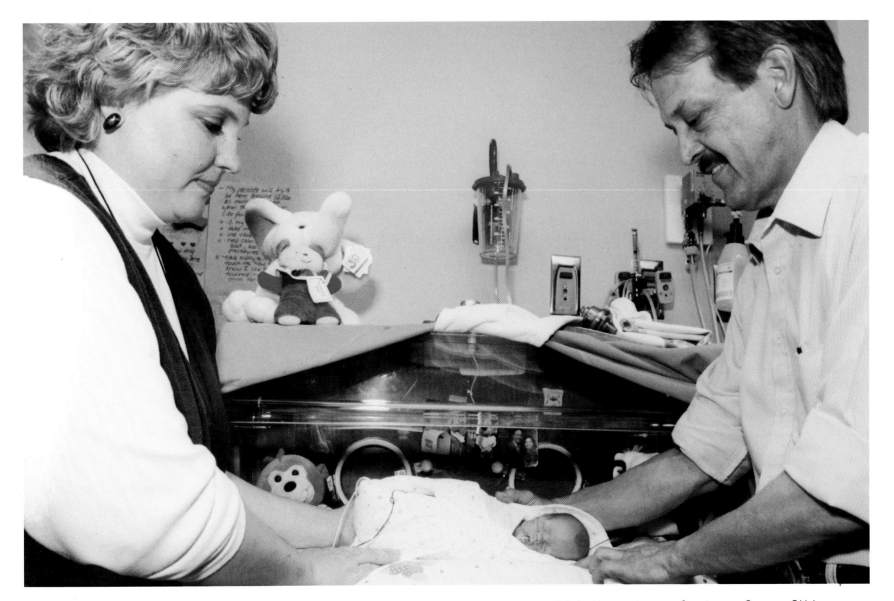

Jaye Hall, nurse manager of the neonatal intensive care unit at Children's Hospital, left, and Gary Whybark soothe Whybark's premature son, Gary, in 1995. *Courtesy Oklahoma Publishing Company.*

against cancer, advances in local heart disease research, and the latest on AIDS research at the OUHSC. The program was sponsored by Macklanburg-Duncan and Boatmen's Bank and was produced by the Presbyterian Health Foundation. In addition to weekly programs, Jayroe often provided health reports for KOCO-TV in Oklahoma City.

One particular program revealed plans for a new Oklahoma clinic for children with cancer. The Jimmy Everest Center for Cancer and Blood Disorders was named for the 17-year-old son of Jim and Christy Everest. In the television program, Jayroe compassionately discussed Jimmy's battle with cancer that resulted in his death in 1992 and the family's plans to turn tragedy into hope through raising funds for a new facility.

PHF made a huge difference in the ability to recruit and pay adequate compensation for leaders of the institutions in the OUHSC. PHF was able to supplement the state salary of Dr. Jay H. Stein when he became senior vice president and provost of OUHSC in 1992. Stein came to OU from the University of Texas Health Science Center in San Antonio and was new on the job when state voters approved a $350 million bond issue that pumped $22.4 million into OUHSC—$4.5 million was for a family practice medicine building and $17.9 million was earmarked for a new biomedical research center.

The total cost of a top quality biomedical research center was anticipated to exceed $45 million. Provost Stein believed a research park on the OHC campus would attract many fine scientists who would develop research programs that would bring large amounts of federal grant money to the campus.

Stein also addressed what continued to be a shortage of primary care physicians in rural Oklahoma. For years, the problem was approached in different ways with no appreciable success. Stein's idea was to cultivate OU medical students' innate altruism to care for people in remote areas and to recruit additional help from high technology, such as building a positron emission tomography (PET scan) facility to house the latest state-of-the-art imaging device.

The key to Stein's plan to place more doctors in rural Oklahoma was to set up a statewide cutting-edge telecommunications and fiber optics system that would link rural hospitals and doctors to big-city medical expertise and advanced diagnostic technology such as PET scans.

While OUHSC officials looked for ways to fund its own biomedical research center, the Presbyterian Health Foundation board of trustees moved forward with plans to build a 26-acre biomedical research park west of Lincoln Boulevard between Northeast 4th and Northeast 8th streets. Reporters were shown the framework of the first building in what would become known as the Presbyterian Health Foundation Research Park. The first structure was a 110,000-square-foot, $6.5 million building.

The need for the research park was recognized by Stanton L. Young and other leaders of the Presbyterian Health Foundation and the Oklahoma Health Center Foundation. Trustees were aware of facilities such as Research Triangle Park in North Carolina connected with Duke University and the University of North Carolina. Young was chairman of the Oklahoma City Urban Renewal Authority and strongly supported the creation of a research park to enhance economic development of the city as medical research expanded and new knowledge was discovered that could be applied for the improvement of human health. To get ideas, Young, Hershel Lamirand, Dennis McGrath, and other leaders toured research parks in Massachusetts and Maryland.

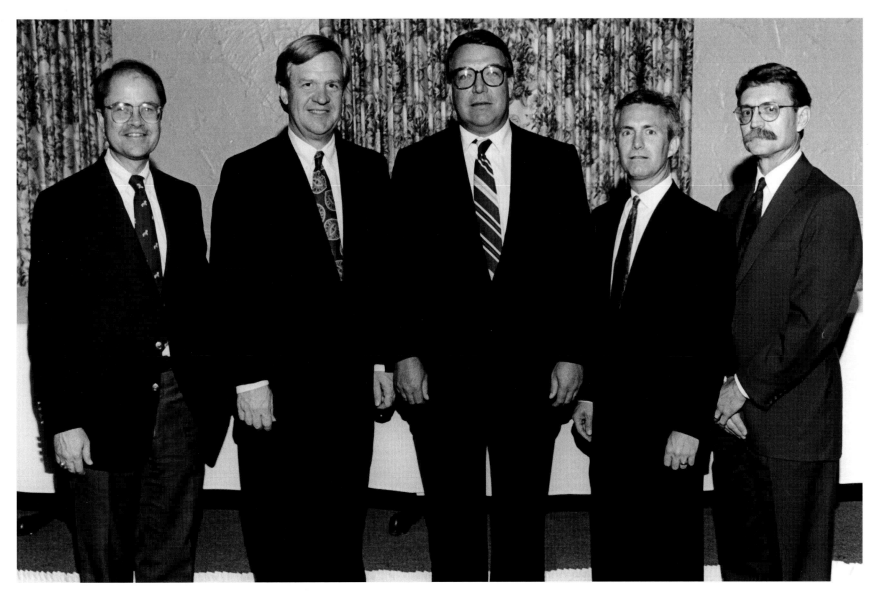

Members of the Oklahoma Medical Research Foundation board of directors in 1992, included, left to right, Dr. J.B. Pratt, Gerald Gamble, Michael A. Cawley, John Mark Paschal, and Dr. Richard Allgood. *Courtesy Oklahoma Publishing Company.*

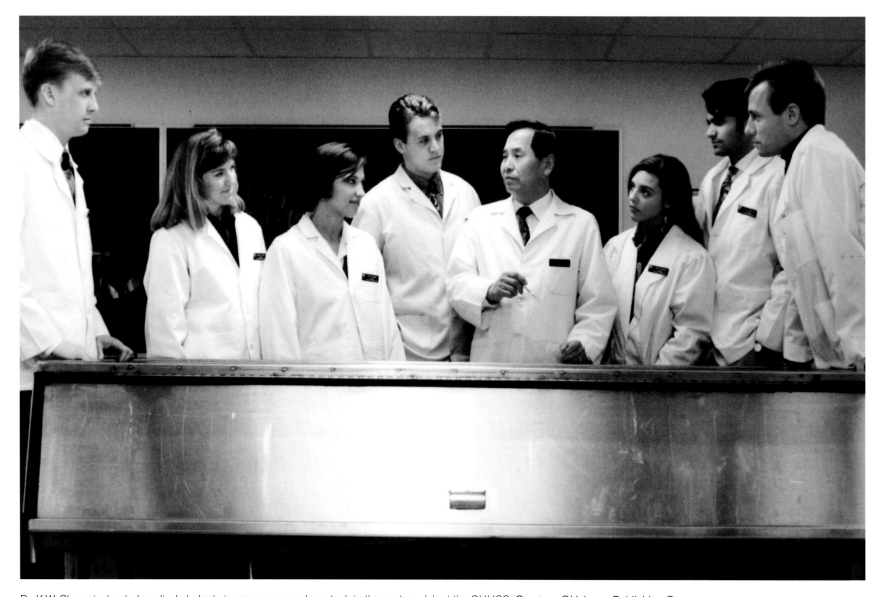

Dr. K.W. Chung instructed medical students in 1995 over a cadaver tank in the anatomy lab at the OUHSC. *Courtesy Oklahoma Publishing Company.*

The idea for a research park was applauded by Dr. William L. "Bill" Parry, chairman of the OU Department of Urology. Research in Parry's department played a major role in jump-starting the development of the research park.

In the beginning the research park was called the Oklahoma Health Center Research Park. At a breakfast briefing of city and state leaders in October, 1994, PHF chairman Stanton L. Young said the research park would offer a place where biomedical discoveries made at OUHSC and OMRF could evolve and develop into new Oklahoma companies that provide services or manufacture products. It was a tremendous boost for the Oklahoma economy, a point recognized by Oklahoma Governor David Walters who presented Young a $500,000 check from the United States Department of Energy to assist with the project.

For many years, hospitals, colleges, and other institutions located in the Oklahoma Health Center drafted and re-drafted emergency plans and conducted disaster drills. What they learned from those drills was tested on April 19, 1995.

At 9:02 a.m., a yellow Ryder rental truck filled with a fertilizer bomb parked in front of the Alfred P. Murrah Federal Building in downtown Oklahoma City and exploded. When the dust from the horrendous explosion settled, 168 people were dead and hundreds more injured. It was the worst act of domestic terrorism in the history of the United States.

Hershel Lamirand, OU Director of University of Affairs, was parking his Nissan Pathfinder in the lot south of the Robert M. Bird Health Sciences Library when the explosion occurred. He looked downtown toward the deafening sound and saw a huge billow of black smoke, dust, and debris rising into the air. Curious, Lamirand raced down Sixth Street toward the Murrah Building. He parked a block from the scene and ran to the north side of the Murrah Building and saw a flood of injured people walking and running from parts of the building that had not been destroyed.

As fire trucks and police cars began to arrive, Lamirand overcame the shock of the tragedy and began calling hospitals in the Oklahoma Health Center, warning them that surely many patients would be headed their way.

It was sheer chaos in the block around the Murrah Building. Hundreds of people were in shock. Most were covered with their own blood or from the blood of other workers who were cut by flying glass and debris from the explosion.

If a disaster had to occur, it was the right time for the availability of medical care. Many physicians were making morning rounds at the five hospitals within a mile of the Murrah Building. When he heard the explosion, Dr. Andy Sullivan went to the top of University Hospital and could see that a downtown building had exploded.

A disaster drill was commenced immediately and operating rooms were cleared of anyone who could be moved. Elective surgeries were canceled. Dr. Sullivan said, "We were ready."

Patients came by ambulance, personal car, and on foot. Dr. Sullivan and Dr. David Tuggle, both pediatric specialists, triaged patients and sent the more serious ones to surgery. Two hours after the explosion, traffic in the University Hospital emergency room slowed to a trickle so Sullivan and Tuggle headed for the Murrah Building. It was a scene of mass confusion as rescue workers dug through huge piles of debris looking for the dead and those who remained alive.

Just after noon, a young woman who had been in the federal building to obtain a Social Security card for her baby was found

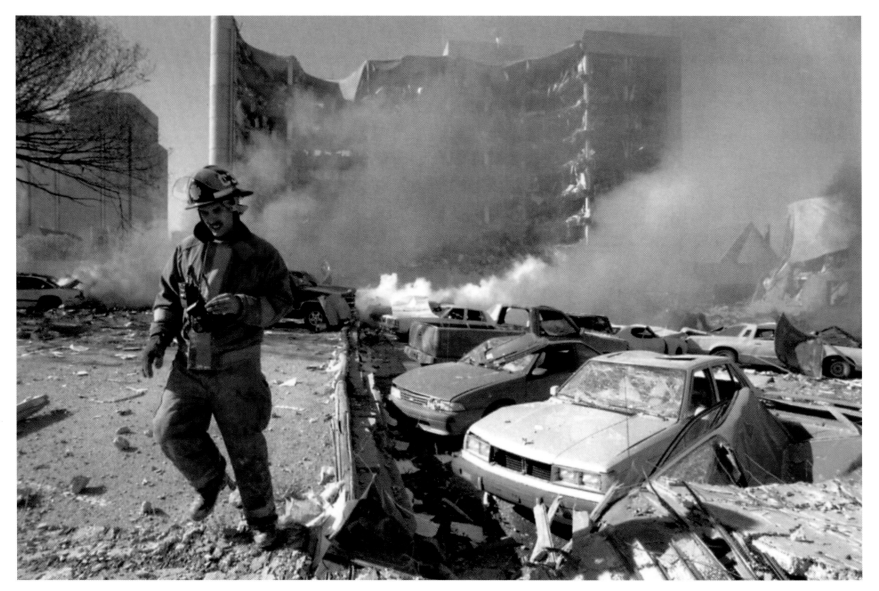

Photographer Jim Argo captured the horrific aftermath of the bombing of the Alfred P. Murrah Federal Building in Oklahoma City on the morning of April 19, 1995.
Courtesy Oklahoma Publishing Company.

trapped in the basement. Daina Bradley was alive but her leg was pinned between two large slabs of concrete. Dr. Sullivan, who had returned to University Hospital to help out in the emergency room, grabbed an amputation kit that contained scalpels, knives, and clamps. As he was leaving, he used his pocketknife to cut a piece of nylon rope that he would be able to use as a tourniquet.

When Sullivan and Tuggle arrived at the Murrah Building, they were led into the dark and smoke-filled basement. They made their way around large pieces of concrete and avoided electrical lines strewn throughout the rubble. For hours, the young woman had laid in six inches of water and was in shock. Sullivan removed his hard hat and crawled on his stomach until he reached her. A light bulb rigged by rescue workers provided a glimmer of light.

Sullivan cleared the rubble from around Bradley's leg and began to tie a tourniquet. Then, news came that a second bomb was in the building and the doctors were ordered to leave. It was gut-wrenching because the woman screamed, "Please don't leave me to die!" Sullivan promised he would return.

After no second bomb materialized, Sullivan again crawled into the small space and tied a rescue harness to the woman's body so she could be pulled from the rubble once he amputated her leg. Sullivan gave the woman medicine to help her forget what was about to happen and prayed that she would not bleed to death and die in his arms as he performed the crude surgery.

The first, second, and third scalpel blades broke as the woman screamed and thrashed about with her free arms and leg. The doctor used his body to pin her leg against the concrete wall and switched to an amputation knife. When hitting against the concrete dulled the knife, he had to finish the job with his pocketknife.

The amputation complete, Bradley was lifted from the rubble,

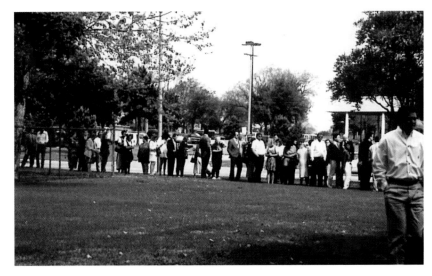

The Oklahoma Blood Institute received an unprecedented response for blood donations following the Murrah Building bombing. *Courtesy Oklahoma Blood Institute.*

survived, and was later fitted with a prosthetic device. Today she lives a normal life. Dr. Sullivan was only one of hundreds of heroes among the thousands of workers at the Oklahoma Health Center who provided care for victims of the Murrah Building bombing that day.

The emergency plan at Children's Hospital also worked unbelievably well. Dr. Terrence Stull remembered, "At one point in the emergency room, I turned around and saw three people standing with clip-boards, numbering all the victims and writing down a description of them. As the families came in, they were matching these descriptions with family statements. One family came in looking for a child in a Barney tee-shirt. A few moments later, parents and child were reunited."

Within ten minutes of the explosion and news of mass casualties, the Oklahoma Blood Institute (OBI) went into action. The OBI had occupied its headquarters in the Oklahoma Health Center since 1982 in a building constructed primarily by funds donated by shopping cart inventor Sylvan Goldman.

With news of the bombing, OBI began delivering blood to area hospitals. Within five hours, hundreds of units of blood were used to keep victims alive. The call went out to the community that more blood would be needed. Hundreds of volunteers arrived. More than 4,700 units of blood were drawn during the first 24 hours after the bombing. Within a three-day period, 7,500 units of blood were drawn, compared to the normal production of 10,000 units in a month.

Another tenant of OHC had a gigantic task related to the Murrah Building Bombing. The Office of the Oklahoma State Medical Examiner had to examine and care for the bodies of the 168 fatalities. It took rescuers several days to remove the bodies from the bombed-out building. It was a massive job. Ray Blakeney, director of operations of the Medical Examiner's office, oversaw the recovery and identification of bodies, setting up the morgue, which included preserving evidence that would later be used in criminal trials, and operation of a family assistance center.

The small Medical Examiner's staff of 32 ballooned to 300, supplemented by many volunteers and staff members of OUHSC. A group of pathologists and dentists helped Medical Examiner personnel examine and identify bodies. Nearly 200 radiology technicians at OHC hospitals took full-body x-rays of each victim. Refrigerated trailers were provided by the Federal Emergency Management Administration (FEMA) for the storage of bodies.

Other members of the OHC provided help in the aftermath of the disaster. The Oklahoma County Chapter of the American Red Cross, from its building at Northeast 6th Street and Lincoln Boulevard, and personnel from the Oklahoma Department of Mental Health staffed the family assistance center set up at First Christian Church.

Red Cross workers responded to the Murrah Building immediately after the explosion to provide first aid and other victim assistance. Red Cross workers parked their trucks as close to the disaster scene as possible and began to help firefighters, police, and other emergency personnel direct the injured to particular hospitals and send families to the right facility where their loved ones were being treated.

Red Cross volunteers served meals to rescue workers. Debby Hampton, who was in charge of volunteers at the Red Cross office in OHC, was overwhelmed with the army of volunteers who had no previous Red Cross experience or training. In the first 24 hours, 1,200 volunteer applications were processed. Judges, lawyers, and doctors helped process applications. Instant training was provided as Red Cross officials made identification tags to allow the volunteers access to the scene of the disaster. In the 30 days following the bombing, the local Red Cross processed 9,400 volunteers. One man even flew from Australia to help. Another man was utilized as a runner, carrying messages and supplies from a soft drink warehouse to the Murrah Building. At the end of one day, he handed Debby Hampton a check for $10,000 made out to the Red Cross.

Years after the dark days of April, 1995, Medical Examiner Office operations director Blakeney reflected, "We absolutely could not have done our job without the people in the Oklahoma Health Center. It was a demonstration of this complex coming together and working together."

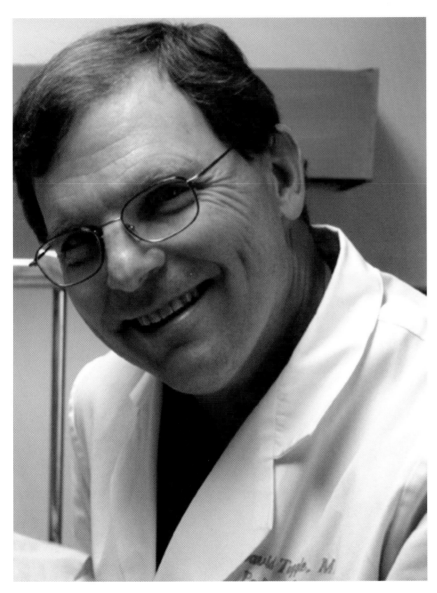

Orthopedic surgeon Dr. David Tuggle was in the rubble of the Murrah Building with Dr. Andy Sullivan, saving the life of a young lady whose leg had to be amputated. *Courtesy University of Oklahoma.*

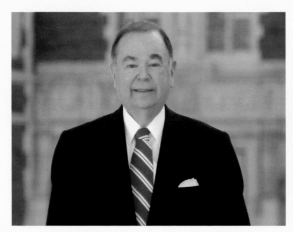
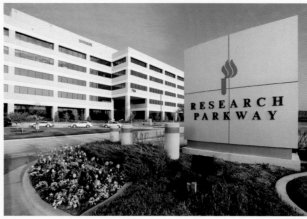
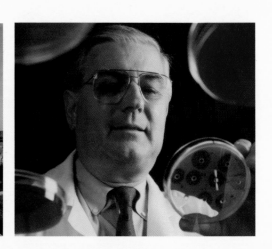

Chapter Six

Building for Research

Research was finally the "name of the game" in the growth and development of the Oklahoma Health Center. The OU College of Medicine, the Oklahoma Medical Research Foundation, the Dean A. McGee Eye Institute, and the Veterans Affairs Medical Center were engaged in biomedical research.

There was a wide area of basic scientific investigation underway on campus. The biggest change in the 1980s and early 1990s was in molecular biology and its application to medicine and biotechnology. Nationwide, the biotech business was beginning to unleash its tremendous potential on economic growth.

The National Institutes of Health (NIH) is a main source of grants funding research in academic health centers such as OUHSC. Dr. John Sokatch, a longtime faculty member, believed that a "good part of a physician's job" should be clinical research. Sokatch described the funding problem faced by researchers, "There is some money available from pharmaceutical companies, but it must be directed toward the kind of research they want to do. To attract any kind of private money, the research must be specifically targeted toward a particular end, such as curing some kind of cancer."

Sokatch taught classes and monitored laboratory work of medical students while allocating time in his schedule to conduct and oversee scientific investigation. In 1995 he was studying gene regulation in bacteria.

In August, 1995, ground was broken by OU President David Boren and other state and university officials for the long-awaited Biomedical Research Center of the OUHSC to be built on Northeast 10th Street west of Stonewall Avenue, across from the Oklahoma Department of Health. More than $8 million in private donations matched $17.9 million in state bond money. At the groundbreaking, Dr. Joseph Ferretti, interim provost of the OU campus in Oklahoma City, said research at OUHSC had increased by more than 250 percent in the previous eight years, although the campus had not gained any new laboratory space since 1976.

Ferretti said, "The Biomedical Research Center will allow us to continue to recruit premier scientists to Oklahoma as well as provide the needed space for already ongoing programs."

Construction of the 105,000-square-foot building took two years. The first floor was designed to contain core laboratories, a seminar room, large conference room, and utility space. The second, third, and fourth floors housed additional laboratories along with offices for principal investigators and shared laboratory support spaces. Activity in the research center created 800 jobs and an estimated $38 million annual impact to the Oklahoma City economy.

At the time the Biomedical Research Center was being built, construction began on a new student union for the OUHSC campus. The 26,000-square-foot building cost $4.3 million. Construction workers completed the Jimmy Everest Center, an addition to Children's Memorial Hospital, in 1995. In other parts of the OHC campus, construction cranes and sounds of table saws and nail guns permeated the air. The Presbyterian Hospital Center for Healthy Living was completed in 1995.

Significant growth to research at OHC came as the Presbyterian Health Foundation saw the opportunity of jump-starting the PHF Research Park by constructing the first building. The challenge was to construct a building as quickly as possible for UroCor, a biomedical company specializing in clinical diagnostic services for urologists. The company chose Oklahoma City for its headquarters even though it had been offered free office space in a research park in Houston, Texas.

Backers of the PHF Research Park on the OHC campus recognized that providing reasonable rent on space built for biomedical laboratory research was a key in attracting companies such as UroCor. The company was formerly known as CytoDiagnostics, Inc., a company formed in Oklahoma City in 1985 by urology professor Dr. George H. Hemstreet.

PHF hired an architect, and a week later employed a contractor. A site plan was developed to accommodate nine buildings. If the project turned out to be successful, it would mean PHF could nurture its first technology transfer from research on the OUHSC campus to commercialization. It was an exciting time.

In September, 1995, Governor Frank Keating joined UroCor President William Hagstrom and other officials to dedicate the $10 million UroCor Building in the PHF Research Park. Dennis McGrath of the Presbyterian Health Foundation told reporters that the milestone in development of the park would make it easier for new science technologies developed by faculty at the OUHSC to make the transition from the academic setting to the marketplace.

UroCor's Hagstrom said, "Two key factors in fostering biotech growth are the availability of space specifically designed for biotechnology application and the desire of state and local government to proactively nurture its development. By developing this research park, Oklahoma has taken an important step in building a real presence."

State government also began to actively provide incentives for private sector involvement in the PHF Research Park. The Oklahoma Center for Advancement of Science and Technology (OCAST), authorized by the legislature in 1987, stepped up its efforts to attract private investments and federal funding.

OCAST used a process known as leverage—leveraging resources to attract top scientists, stimulate development, and achieve measurable economic impact in the state. As the state's technology-based economic development agency, OCAST had its beginnings during the bad economic times of the mid-1980s, but survived budget cuts to establish itself as a major player in investing in research, development, technology commercialization, and manufacturing modernization.

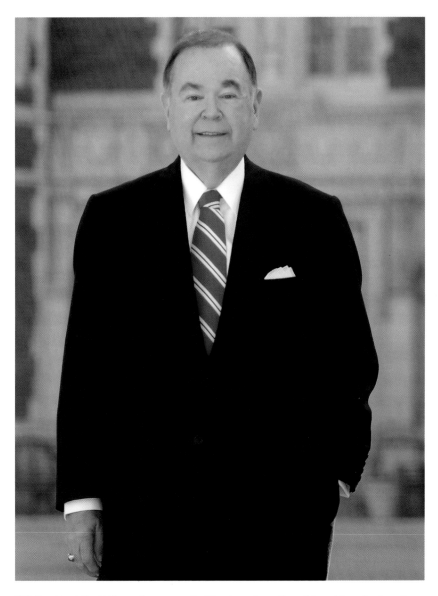

OU President David Boren has supported the transformation of the old medical center area to a world-class health care campus since his term as governor in the 1970s. As United States Senator, he assisted OHC officials in obtaining federal assistance. As president of OU, his leadership has resulted in record fund raising and expenditures on the OUHSC campus. *Courtesy University of Oklahoma.*

Oklahoma's Crown Jewel

In the mid-1990s, the winds of change recaptured the imaginations of university leaders who embraced an opportunity to transform the landscape of this 300-acre campus into a booming biomedical magnet that drives financial security and no longer is satisfied with being the "best kept secret in Oklahoma."

As one of only four comprehensive academic health centers in the nation, the University of Oklahoma Health Sciences Center offers an exciting opportunity for some of the nation's best researchers to investigate new ideas in the laboratory while students learn about disease and the human condition first-hand in the clinic.

More than 600 physicians are receiving residency training for more than 40 specialties and sub-specialties in Oklahoma City and Tulsa. In addition to training physicians, the OU Health Sciences Center serves as the state's training facility for physician's assistants, biomedical scientists, nurses, dentists, pharmacists and a wide range of allied health and public health professionals, including nutritional specialists, radiation therapists, physical and occupational therapists, public health policy specialists and environmental health specialists.

The OU Health Sciences Center serves more than 3,900 students in more than 70 graduate and undergraduate programs in Oklahoma City and at the Schusterman Center at OU-Tulsa. It has strengthened its partnerships with private donors and foundations such as the Presbyterian Health Foundation and the University Hospitals Authority and Trust to attract the best and brightest scientists, physicians, students and other health professionals to Oklahoma City through endowments and unequalled opportunities. With a core in place, leaders are building a network of excellence for research, education and patient care that has had and will continue to have a far-reaching impact like no other place in Oklahoma.

Central to this recent growth has been the creation, funding and construction of the $210 million OU Cancer Institute, which will soon become the only cancer center in Oklahoma designated as a comprehensive cancer center by the National Cancer Institute.

Since 1996, new construction worth more than $600 million in capital improvements has included a new student union, two state-of-the-art biomedical research facilities, the Harold Hamm Oklahoma Diabetes Center, the $27 million OU Physicians Building and a new 114,000-square-foot College of Allied Health for training the next generation of health professionals.

The investment has helped triple the amount of research funding received by the OU Health Sciences Center in the last 10 years to more than $150 million, including $53 million from the National Institutes of Health – considered the gold standard for research – to address research projects ranging from cancer and environmental issues to vision and dental health. The OU Health Sciences Center ranks tenth nationally in vision research funding from the NIH and fifteenth nationally in NIH funding for microbiology.

The investment and growth also has spurred creation of Presbyterian Research Park to the west, which not only houses more laboratory space for scientists, but has attracted and nurtured dozens of biomedical businesses with commercial products developed from research at the OU Health Sciences Center and other entities on campus. And, the potential is enormous. The current growth has been achieved with just 15 percent of overall funding coming from the state. Health leaders are hopeful that future investment by the state to fund the health sciences center at the national average would produce an invaluable return and spark a biomedical boom.

All of this effort in education, research and patient care has built the University of Oklahoma Health Sciences Center into the state's premier academic health center and a regional leader in meeting the challenges of 21st-century health care where solutions will bring healthier tomorrows for all Oklahomans.

Dr. Joseph J. Ferretti
Senior Vice President and Provost
University of Oklahoma Health Sciences Center

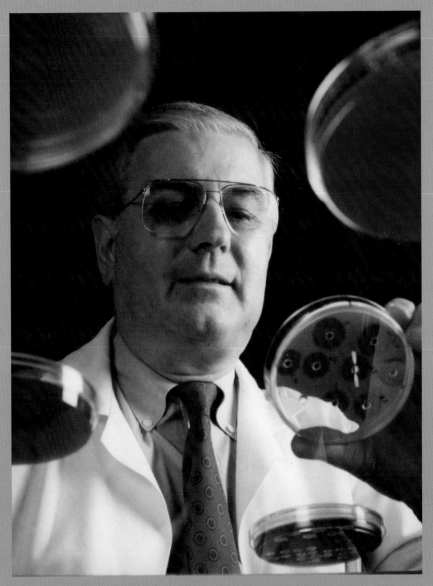

Dr. Joseph J. Ferretti is Provost of the OU Health Sciences Center and a major player in the growth of the Oklahoma Health Center. *Courtesy Oklahoma Publishing Company.*

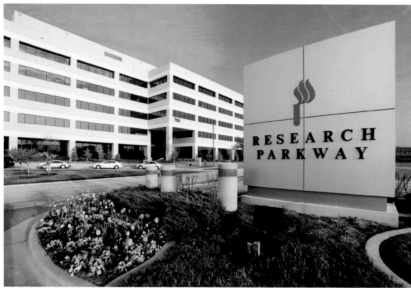

The Presbyterian Health Foundation is the guiding hand behind the world-class PHF Research Park. *Courtesy Presbyterian Health Foundation.*

By 2009, OCAST had spent nearly $200 million to attract more than $2.8 billion in private investment and federal funding.

To foster innovation in existing and developing businesses, OCAST supports basic and applied research, facilitates technology transfer between research laboratories and commercial companies, provides seed capital for new innovative firms and their products, and encourages competition in national and international markets by small and medium-sized Oklahoma manufacturing firms.

In response to OCAST's initiative to establish a center to support technology commercialization, i2E was created in 1997. As a private, not-for-profit corporation, i2E focuses on wealth creation by growing the technology-based entrepreneurial economy in Oklahoma. To accomplish its objectives, i2E provides technology development knowledge and know-how, delivers comprehensive enterprise development services, and helps new companies stay viable. i2e supports new advanced technology companies from proof-of-concept through early market entry.

The state also funded the Oklahoma Technology Commercialization Center (OTCC) which has worked with public and private technology experts to assist researchers, inventors, entrepreneurs, and companies turn high-tech start-up companies into exceptional business opportunities in Oklahoma. OTCC is operated by i2E.

In January, 1997, OUHSC officials unveiled plans for construction of a $17 million ambulatory care center on the campus. Associate Provost and Dean of the College of Medicine Jerry Vannatta said the center was needed because the medical clinics operated by OUHSC were spread out in different locations and confused both patients and doctors. The 120,000-square-foot facility was intended to be used by hundreds of university-affiliated physicians and thousands of patients each year. Vannatta said, "Our clinics are difficult to find. They are neither patient-friendly nor doctor-friendly." When completed, the highly-visible, easily-accessible center predictably met the teaching and practice needs of the faculty in the OU College of Medicine.

The mid-1990s brought yet another crisis for University and Children's hospitals and the OU College of Medicine. Since shortly after statehood, both hospitals, with the help of skilled faculty and residents from the medical school, had provided the bulk of hospital care for citizens from all corners of the state who had no insurance or who were eligible for some type of public assistance, or later, Medicaid benefits.

Income from Medicaid-eligible patients comprised 46 percent

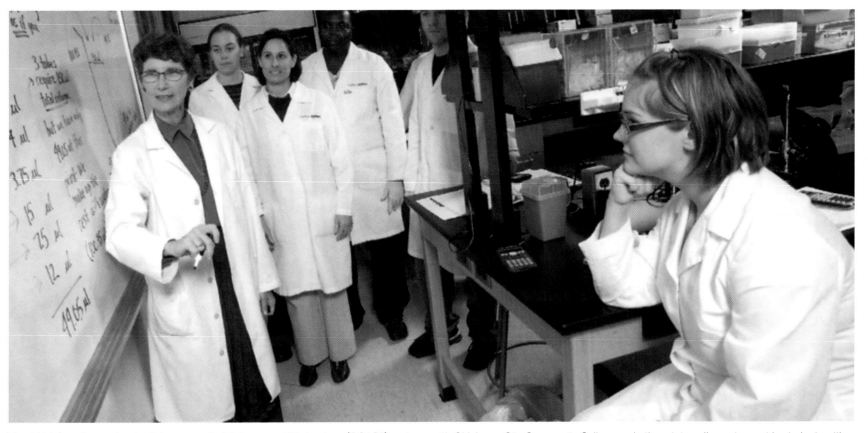

The Oklahoma Center for the Advancement of Science and Technology (OCAST) partners with Oklahoma City Community College and other state colleges to provide students with on-the-job training while working toward their associate's degree in biotechnology. *Courtesy OCAST.*

of University Hospital's $150 million income. However, when the legislature converted Medicaid, a federal-state program that buys medical services for the poor, to a managed care system, University and Children's hospitals were placed in jeopardy. All hospitals in the state suffered loss of income, but no institution had as much Medicaid participation as University and Children's. Officials knew that in other states where Medicaid programs had changed to managed care, academic medical centers such as OHC lost 50 percent of their patients.

After four HMOs won bids for SoonerCare, the state's new, prepaid, managed-care Medicaid system that began operation on July 1, 1995, University and Children's began piling up huge deficits. Even with the elimination of 600 positions and closing the O'Donoghue Rehabilitation Center, there was still a shortfall in the hospitals' budgets.

In October, 1995, headlines in *The Oklahoma Observer*, "University Hospital on Endangered List," told the story. With reduced income, University and Children's hospitals had a budget deficit. The state legislature did not have enough surplus funds to even begin to solve the problem. Legislators and university and hospital administrators hinted of the possibility of closing both University and Children's hospitals.

Closing the hospitals would be bad enough, but without the hospitals, College of Medicine leaders feared sending their students and faculty to learn and teach in other hospitals in the area would endanger the medical school's accreditation. There was no doubt closure of the hospitals would hurt Oklahoma's reputation, and the state's remaining hospitals would be forced to take up the slack in providing care for indigent or uninsured citizens.

Leaders looked for a solution. Consultants were hired to evaluate the Oklahoma City area and determine if too many hospital beds existed, a common perception of civic leaders. Veteran corporate and association representative Clayton Taylor was hired to manage the consultants and provide a central point for gathering information about the problem.

Once the consultants completed their assessment, it was determined that Oklahoma City truly did have too many hospital beds. Some observers quietly suggested that the only answer was to close University and Children's and stop the bleeding of red ink. However, OU President David Boren, leaders of the legislature, OUHSC officials, and major partners in the OHC complex decided to look for other alternatives. There were too many negative repercussions that would

no doubt impact the entire state should the two hospitals close.

Consultants found that many non-indigent patients in Oklahoma would not use University or Children's because they perceived the two as welfare hospitals. The general public was not aware of the progress being made to raise the level of research and patient care. Anyone who actually ended up in the hospitals sang their praises—but the masses of people in the state still clung to their long-held beliefs that quality medical care had to be sought someplace else besides University and Children's hospitals.

Taylor remembered, "Everyone agreed we could not let the hospitals close. No upper-tier medical school in the nation operated in a decentralized situation. The finest medical training was taking place in cities where the medical school was but a few steps from leading patient care facilities."

When it was obvious that state money would not be available to fix the problem, hospital and state officials investigated leasing the hospitals. Proposals were sent to the nation's major health care corporations, but the answer lay less than a block away, at the door of Columbia/HCA, the owner of Presbyterian Hospital.

University and Children's hospitals already had taken steps to move their administration into a new era. In 1993, the state legislature took control of both hospitals from the Department of Human Services and placed them under the authority of the University Hospitals Authority, a six-person board comprised of one appointee of the governor, the State Senate, the State House of Representatives, the director of DHS, and the Provost of the OUHSC. The CEO of University Hospitals was designated as an ex-officio, non-voting member. The first members of the University Hospital Authority were Macklanburg-Duncan President Mike Samis; Tulsa County Medical Society director Paul Patton; Tulsa attorney Dean Luthey; Dr. Garth Splinter, director of the Oklahoma Health Care Authority; OUHSC Provost Dr. Jay Stein; and University Hospitals CEO Dr. Andy Lasser.

Columbia/HCA, which became Columbia Health Corporation, was the nation's largest hospital company and expressed great interest in adding the management of University and Children's hospitals to its ownership of Presbyterian Hospital.

In November, 1995, a partnership between Columbia, University and Children's hospitals, and the faculty and administration of the OU College of Medicine was announced. Dean Luthey, chairman of the Oklahoma Hospitals Authority board, told reporters that Columbia was the only potential partner to save the hospitals. The deal required Columbia to give $50 million to be split between the hospital trust and the OUHSC.

Under the terms of the original agreement, Columbia would manage the hospitals under the watchful eye of a ten-man board, five from the Hospital Authority and five representing Columbia. The state would retain ownership of the property. Cash flow would be split—60 percent for Columbia and 40 percent for the trust.

From the outset, it was apparent the lease arrangement with Columbia would save huge appropriations for capital expenditures at University and Children's, and, most importantly, assure that the hospitals would remain open. During negotiations over the next three years, legislators weighed in on the importance of University and Children's continuing to provide indigent care to Oklahomans. Some legislative leaders did not like the idea of giving up state control of the hospitals, but time has proven their decision to do so was correct.

College of Medicine Dean Jerry Vannatta, who grew up on a wheat farm in the Oklahoma Panhandle, became the quarterback in the massive effort to make the partnership with Columbia work. He fully accepted what consultants for the State Senate, State House of Representatives, and OUHSC had concluded—University and Children's hospitals could not survive without a capital partner. Dr. Donald Halverstadt called the relationship between Columbia and OUHSC the "single greatest opportunity" he had seen on the campus in his 29 years.

In early 1997, the long-awaited completion of negotiations of the partnership between Columbia, the University Hospitals Authority, and the OUHSC materialized. It had been a complicated process that concluded in a lease agreement of more than 400 pages. David Dunlap, president of the Oklahoma division of Columbia, led the effort for his company. Several legislators paid close attention to details of the agreement and supported the deal. Significant contributions came from House members such as Jari Askins of Duncan, now Oklahoma's lieutenant governor; Calvin Anthony of Stillwater, a graduate of the OU College of Pharmacy; and Jim Hamilton of Poteau, chairman of the House Appropriations Committee.

In the State Senate, President Pro Tempore Stratton Taylor of Claremore, Ben Robinson of Muskogee, and Glenn Coffee of Oklahoma City championed the passing of management of the hospitals to Columbia. Dr. Joseph Ferretti, Dr. Jerry Vannatta, and Dr. Dewayne Andrews played pivotal roles in guiding negotiations for the OUHSC. Sean Burrage, an aide to OU President Boren, kept his boss fully informed on progress of the elongated negotiations. The partnership had long been envisioned by Boren. In 1977, when he was governor, he drew a rough sketch of what an expanded Oklahoma Health Center might look like some day.

Ron Yordi, chairman of the Oklahoma Health Center

Foundation, led his board in supporting both the concept and the final plan. Civic leader Stanton L. Young, as usual, spent many hours talking to legislators, state officials, and business leaders about the advantages of the agreement with Columbia.

The final agreement between Columbia and the University Hospitals Authority survived a test in the Oklahoma Supreme Court and won approval of state legislative leaders and officials of other parties. In essence, the agreement provided:

1. Columbia would operate both University and Children's hospitals. The state would retain ownership of the teaching hospitals and Presbyterian would remain the property of Columbia;

2. The three hospitals would be jointly governed by a ten-member board—five members representing the University Hospitals Authority and five representing Columbia. The Authority chairman would chair the new board;

3. Revenues from Presbyterian, University, and Children's would be co-mingled, with Columbia receiving 70 percent of the profits and the Authority getting 30 percent;

4. All hospital employees would remain or become Columbia employees;

5. Colombia would contribute $50 million, with $26 million going to the OU College of Medicine and $24 million to the University Hospitals Authority to update facilities and equipment.

As if the complicated lease-management arrangement needed additional hurdles, news of Columbia being investigated for Medicare fraud in 1997 caused some legislators to want to halt the deal. Leaders who had hammered out details of the arrangement had to ignore the rumblings of wrongdoing. On July 22, 1997,

the OU Board of Regents put its final stamp of approval on the agreement. President Boren said, "The choice is not pleasant. Either form a partnership with Columbia, who had been a good citizen despite being investigated for misdealing with Medicaid, or let the state's largest teaching hospitals sink under financial pressure."

"Let us Pray for a Good Marriage" was the title of an article in the monthly journal of the Oklahoma County Medical Society, whose president, Dr. John Bozalis, hoped that the unprecedented marriage of state functions to care for the poor and uninsured, support the medical school and teaching hospitals, and the privatization of the hospitals' management would work.

Looking back, leasing University and Children's hospitals to Columbia was a brilliant move. Clayton Taylor said, "Whatever the OU College of Medicine and the teaching hospitals have become today, would not happened without the addition of Columbia as a capital partner." Oklahoma Governor Frank Keating gave the agreement its highest accolade. Keating said, "It is the greatest successful example of privatization of a government service."

The Columbia and University Hospitals Authority agreement is still considered a model arrangement in the world of health care. Stanton L. Young said, "It has been an incredibly successful partnership for Oklahoma and its people."

University Hospitals Authority and Trust

Created by Oklahoma's Legislature in 1993, the University Hospitals Authority assumed responsibility for the University Hospital and the Children's Hospital of Oklahoma and their related clinics, known jointly as the "University Hospitals." For a variety of reasons, including drastic changes that occurred in the healthcare landscape by the mid-1990s, the university hospitals were experiencing enormous financial problems. Their survival was uncertain. No medical school can survive and prosper without a vibrant and successful teaching hospital closely affiliated with it. Consequently, the future of medical education and residency training, the care of large segments of our state's population, and much of the biomedical research in Oklahoma was in doubt and facing a potential crisis.

In far-reaching action, the Legislature created the University Hospitals Trust in 1997, with the members of the Authority serving as the trustees of the Trust. This was a bold move, allowing far greater latitude for needed changes and business practices than authorized for the Authority. By 1998, the Joint Operating Agreement for the new management of the University Hospitals and the Presbyterian Hospital under one umbrella structure and governance had been formed, this entity ultimately to become known as the OU Medical Center. This venture merged the interests of the State (represented through the Trust), the University of Oklahoma, and HCA into a unique partnership to ensure the future of our major teaching hospitals and the medical school.

The subsequent story of the JOA and the University Hospital Trust is nothing short of astonishing. Turning millions of dollars of annually recurring hospital deficits into a sound business operation with a reasonable margin provided the catalyst needed to sustain operations and launch major developments in the OU Medical Center, in the College of Medicine and in the Health Sciences Center.

Through its participation in the joint venture, its use of innovative financing mechanisms, and by taking advantage of designated state-federal matching programs, the University Hospitals Trust since 1998 has provided over $77 million in capital related expenditures in support of the College of Medicine and Health Sciences Center. Moreover, the Trust has invested $65 million in research and education grants for programs involving the HSC colleges. Such notable projects as financing of the OU Physicians medical office building, contributing to the construction of the biomedical research center phase II, providing new equipment for the College of Dentistry, and investment in the Cardiac Arrhythmia Research Institute, now known as the Heart Rhythm Institute, are only a few of the projects that have benefited from the Trust. Now the Trust has set itself to the important task of providing a beautiful, new children's outpatient care center to replace aging and outmoded facilities.

The University Hospitals Authority continues to make every effort to maximize its appropriations by accessing federal matching funds to enhance payments to Oklahoma hospitals and colleges of medicine for the reimbursement of uncompensated care and graduate medical education. Currently the Authority utilizes more than 85% of its appropriations to match and draw federal funds. These programs are administered by the Oklahoma Healthcare Authority and approved by the Center for Medicare and Medicaid Services. These appropriations have been increased significantly by the Oklahoma legislature since the inception of these programs to help meet the growing needs of the Tulsa hospital systems and the academic colleges.

Dean Gandy, Executive Director
University Hospitals Authority and Trust

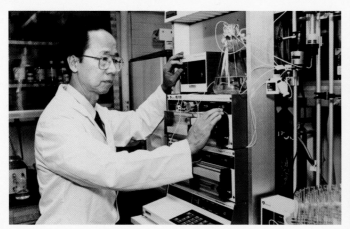 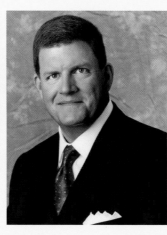 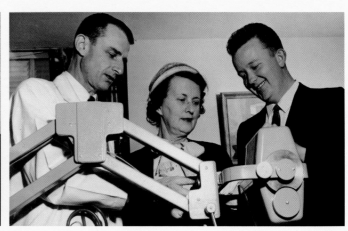

Chapter Seven

Steady Growth

Dr. William G. Thurman retired in 1997 after 18 years as president of the Oklahoma Medical Research Foundation. He was replaced by Dr. J. Donald Capra. The change of leadership came during the year that OMRF was celebrating its 50th anniversary. In some ways, the growth and development of OMRF mirrored the strides the campus of the Oklahoma Health Center was making.

OMRF's home was but a gently sloping, grassy field with shade trees across from University and Children's hospitals when a group of OU College of Medicine alumni began discussing ways to attract medical personnel, especially scientific researchers, to Oklahoma. The doctors found existing facilities for research at the state-run hospitals and the medical school were a significant stumbling block. There was no laboratory space where medical personnel could undertake research.

The idea sparked the creation of an endowment fund to raise money for a medical research institute. OMRF officially was chartered on August 28, 1948. The original stated purpose of the organization was to promote the improvement of human health and well-being by encouraging, fostering, and conducting scientific investigations and education in the sciences. The charter allowed OMRF to conduct research independently or in conjunction with the medical school or other components of the university medical center.

Sir Alexander Fleming, the distinguished British scientist who discovered penicillin, was the featured speaker at the dedication of the original OMRF facility on July 3, 1949. It was a hot Oklahoma day, and Fleming arrived in his customary heavy English wool tweeds. Medical school dean, Dr. Mark Everett, made a hurried trip to a local haberdasher to pick out some lighter-weight clothing for the Nobel Prize winner.

It took only 10 years for OMRF to begin making research history. In 1959, lab assistant Jordan Tang discovered only the second known gastric enzyme. During Bill Thurman's years as president, OMRF scientists had turned much of their attention to molecular biology, as money was raised to expand facilities and

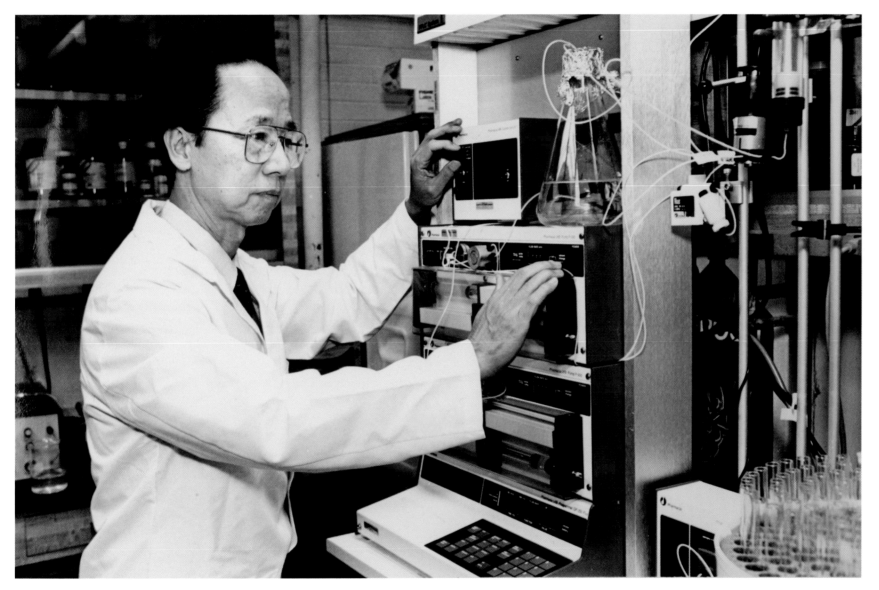

Dr. Jordan Tang shows reporters equipment used in the discovery of a gene that stops the growth of the AIDS virus in human cells in laboratory tests. Tang began making research news at the Oklahoma Medical Research Foundation in the late 1950s. *Courtesy Oklahoma Publishing Company.*

add personnel. Programs in arthritis, immunology, immunobiology, cancer, and protein synthesis were added to basic science research. Much of the federal money for research came from the National Institutes of Health.

Under Thurman's watch, OMRF both competed and cooperated with OUHSC for research dollars. OMRF built central facilities that could be used by researchers at the medical school and the teaching hospitals. A significant step was taken when OMRF joined forces with the Presbyterian Health Foundation to occasionally bring together a small group of scientists to project the future of scientific investigation. Dr. Thurman said, "It was very informal, there were no papers prepared. We just sat around and talked about what's going to happen in the next five or ten years. That, along with our scientific board of visitors, allowed us to clearly address where we were going."

By 1997, OMRF's annual budget was approaching $30 million and recognized as an elite scientific institution. Its new president, Dr. Capra, said, "OMRF can hold its place with the best in the country and the world, ranking with the Salk Institute in California and the Basel Institute in Switzerland." More than half the OMRF budget came from NIH, the American Cancer Society, and the American Heart Association. The remainder of funds came from a wide variety of donors.

OMRF researchers often were honored for their achievements. In 1996, the husband and wife team of Drs. Ronald and Joan Conaway received the Amgen Award for significant work in the application of biochemistry and molecular biology to the understanding of disease. The Conaways were recognized for their work on RNA synthesis for the previous 12 years. They identified a genetic link to acute myeloid leukemia.

Across the OHC campus in the research park, ZymeTX, a research, administrative, and marketing organization, launched a new test for viral influenza in the fall of 1997. The test, known as Virazyme, was patented by OMRF. At the public announcement that three years of laboratory analysis and patent defense had borne fruit, Bill Thurman, Stanton L. Young, Jean Gumerson, and others were honored for their vision. ZymeTX Chief Executive Officer Peter Livingston said, "Oklahoma will someday become a hotbed of biotechnology."

As tenants such as ZymeTX in the first PHF Research Park building were producing results, ground was broken in May, 1997, for a second structure, a $9.2 million building west of the park's first building. The first building, known as the UroCor Building, was 100 percent occupied more than a year ahead of schedule. At the groundbreaking, a healthy future was predicted by Gerald Gamble, Oklahoma City Chamber of Commerce chairman, and Stanton L. Young, who said, "It is probably not more than just a footnote in the history of Oklahoma City, but it is a recognition of the continuation of reaffirmation of a partnership, a very important partnership of the federal, state, and city governments, and the private sector."

The emerging partnerships between scientific research at OUHSC, Dean A. McGee Eye Institute, and the Oklahoma Medical Research Foundation and private companies planning to develop and market the fruits of research, received a shot in the arm with the passage of State Questions 680 and 681 in 1998. The ground work for publicizing the need for the amendments was laid by the Oklahoma Health Center Foundation and the State Chamber. By approving the constitutional amendments, voters cleared the way for state universities and their researchers to form business partnerships

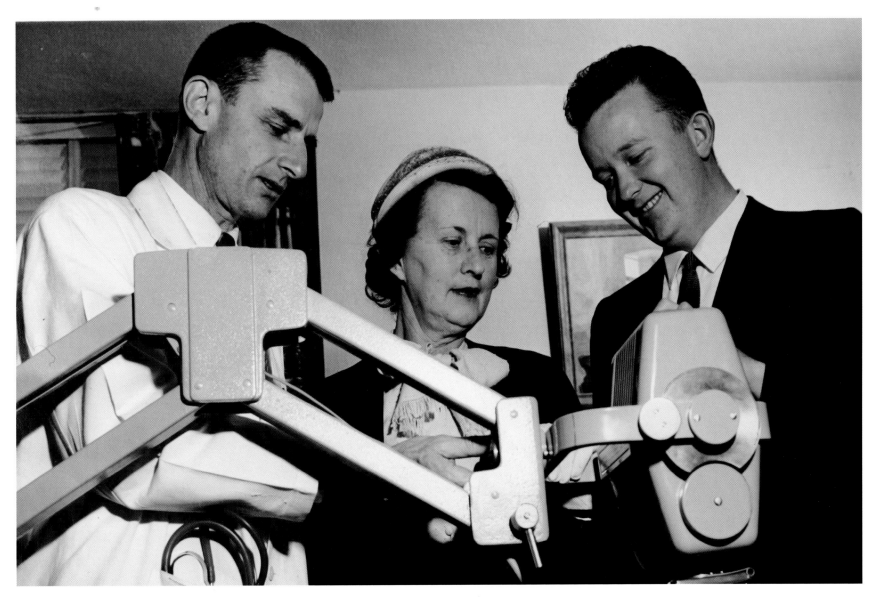

Dr. Leonard P. Eliel, coordinator of research at the Oklahoma Medical Research Foundation, shows Mrs. Donald O. Turner and J.B. Howser, Jr., both of Chandler, a new portable X-ray machine presented to OMRF by the citizens of Chandler in 1950. *Courtesy Oklahoma Publishing Company.*

with private companies. Governor Frank Keating created a cabinet level position of Secretary of Science and Technology.

Also in 1998, leaders of OUHSC gathered to reflect on progress made during the final decade of the twentieth century. The Presbyterian Health Foundation had become the largest single donor to OU, granting more than $35 million since its creation in 1985. The transfer of management of the teaching hospitals to Columbia allowed OUHSC to maintain high standards for medical education, foster an environment where research could grow, and ensure quality patient care.

OUHSC was meeting its charge from the legislature to care for Oklahoma's indigent population. Statistics showed that highly-trained specialists at University and Children's hospitals were providing care for 50 percent of the state's indigent citizens. Family nurse practitioners who completed master's degrees in the OU College of Nursing were helping meet health care needs of rural and medically under-served Oklahomans. A new program prepared pediatric nurse practitioners to serve as school nurses.

The Oklahoma Poison Control Center was operated by the OU College of Pharmacy around the clock to prevent poisonings and manage toxic exposure. The center received more than 60,000 calls in 1997.

The OU College of Medicine was recognized by *U.S. News and World Report* as one of the top 20 comprehensive medical schools in the country. OUHSC is one of only four academic health centers in the nation with seven professional schools—Allied Health, Dentistry, Medicine, Nursing, Pharmacy, Public Health, and Graduate Studies.

OU had become known as one of the primary centers in the world for genome studies, ranking second in the world for the number of microbial genomes being sequenced. The newly completed Stanton L. Young Biomedical Research Center was a state-of-the-art facility integrating the various teaching, clinical, and research components of the seven OUHSC colleges. OU President Boren said, "With this facility, OU will be able to recruit and retain outstanding researchers who will invigorate research efforts and increase research funding."

Other partners in the Oklahoma Health Center reported outstanding milestones. By 1998, Children's Medical Research Institute reached its original goal of endowing five chairs in pediatric research at the OUHSC. But, directors did not rest on their laurels. Instead, they hired a new executive director, Kathy McCracken, and broadened their mission to raise funds to enrich the existing endowed chairs, created new endowed chairs, and provide funding for grants for projects involving medical research for children.

The startling success of the marriage of OUHSC, OMRF, and private companies housed in the PHF Research Park began paying huge dividends. The first major success was Novazyme Pharmaceuticals, Inc., a company created in 1999 based upon research of Dr. William Canfield in his lab at OUHSC. Canfield, one of the world's leading glycobiologists, developed biotherapies for the treatment of lysosomal storage disorders, a group of genetic diseases caused by the absence of certain cellular enzymes.

Novazyme produced a series of novel protein engineering technologies shown in pre-clinical studies to greatly enhance the targeting and uptake of replacement enzymes. In 2001, Novazyme merged with pharmaceutical giant, Genzyme. The Novazyme start-up gave OHC officials great hope for the future.

Also in 1999, Emergent Technologies, Inc. (ETI), a regionally-based venture capital and management services firm, created its first investment fund, Emergent-OU, Ltd., to launch three technologies being researched at the OUHSC. The following year, a second fund was created to make further investments in the first three companies and provided seed capital for other projects.

ETI Pure Protein developed a unique method to produce soluble protein from human cell lines, focusing on the discovery of new targets to prevent and treat infectious disease and cancer. Other ETI-funded companies developed unique capabilities to create several genes from different species of bacteria that synthesized hyaluronic acid, synthesized compounds for the growing anticoagulation market, and developed new technology to produce compounds from bacteria that is more efficient than retrieving the same compounds from other sources such as animal by-products.

With the help of OCAST and PHF, InterGenetics, Incorporated, was established in 1999 to provide momentum for genetic research in cancer risk intervention. Early work that led to a breast cancer risk test began at the Noble Foundation laboratories in the late 1980s, but was moved to OMRF in Oklahoma City in 1993. By 1999, grants from OCAST and PHF allowed the company to obtain patents for its first commercial product, OncoVue Breast Cancer Risk Test, the world's first broad genetic predictive test for breast cancer.

The third building in the PHF Research Park was under construction in 2000 when foundation vice president, Dennis McGrath, told a medical reporter for *The Daily Oklahoman* how important PHF's mission was to support medical research by helping small companies to commercialize medical research. McGrath said, "What we do is provide low-cost space to medical start-up companies that otherwise would not be able to have space.

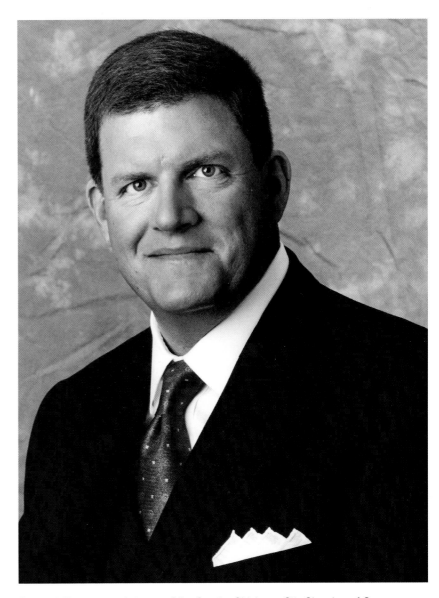

Clayton I. Bennett, as chairman of the Greater Oklahoma City Chamber of Commerce, challenged civic and business leaders to make the Oklahoma Health Center a priority in the development of Oklahoma City. *Courtesy Oklahoma Heritage Association.*

We offer a low-cost alternative to companies that are so young, they couldn't lease space from anybody else." The third PHF Research Park building, at 135,000 square feet, was the largest of the original three buildings.

By 2000, at the dawn of the new century, civic leaders called the world of biotechnology research being conducted on the Oklahoma Health Center campus "a major economic boost." PHF President Jean Gumerson was pleased with new companies taking research developed by scientists at institutions on the OHC campus and making them commercially marketable.

"We are now in the midst of a biological revolution," wrote Dr. Joseph Ferretti, OUHSC Provost, in a 2000 op-ed article in *The Daily Oklahoman.* Ferretti predicted that the study of genomes and new technologies would provide remarkable new tools to improve the quality of human life. Ferretti wrote:

> As a research scientist, it is the future applications of genome information that most intrigue me…With unprecedented knowledge about our own unique genetic makeup, we will be able more than ever before to make wise decisions about our own health… A revolution in pharmacogenomics will allow drugs to be tailored for the individual patient.

The Dean McGee Eye Institute announced a joint venture with NovaMed, a leading eye care services company focused on laser vision correction, in 2000. DMEI president David W. Parke II and his board of directors had made a nationwide search for a reputable laser vision correction sales and marketing partner before choosing NovaMed. The partnership allowed DMEI to at least consider expanding into future markets. DMEI was already the largest eye care center in the Southwest.

Also in 2000, a new research center was established at OUHSC to focus on the role complex carbohydrates play in the health and disease. Dr. Richard Cummings, professor in the OU Department of Biochemistry and Molecular Biology, was named acting director of the Oklahoma Center for Medical Glycobiology, only the third such center in the United States. The new center addressed the needs of Oklahoma researchers at OUHSC and the Oklahoma Medical Research Foundation working in the area of glycobiology.

The year 2000 saw two major announcements at the Oklahoma Health Center regarding diseases that affect many Oklahomans and millions of Americans—diabetes and cancer.

In a landmark partnership agreement, OUHSC and the Choctaw Nation of Oklahoma teamed to combat an emerging diabetes epidemic ravaging the health of Indian children. The agreement allowed specialists from OUHSC to work with some of the nearly 20,000 Choctaw children who suffer from Type-2 Diabetes. The disease is more prevalent in Native Americans than any other group. Dr. Kenneth Copeland, holder of the Paul and Ruth Jonas Chair in Pediatric Diabetes, said the new partnership was part of OU's commitment to enhance health care in the entire state. Copeland led a group of doctors, nutritionists, psychologists, and others from OU to visit health clinics in areas of southeast Oklahoma where the largest concentration of Choctaws live.

Plans were unveiled in 2000 to build a world-class cancer treatment center on the OUHSC campus. OU Regents and OU President Boren said the $210 million center would provide a central location for cancer research, treatment, and education. Provost Ferretti pointed out that Oklahomans have one of the highest death rates in the nation from cancer and other diseases related to smoking, yet Oklahoma was the only state in the

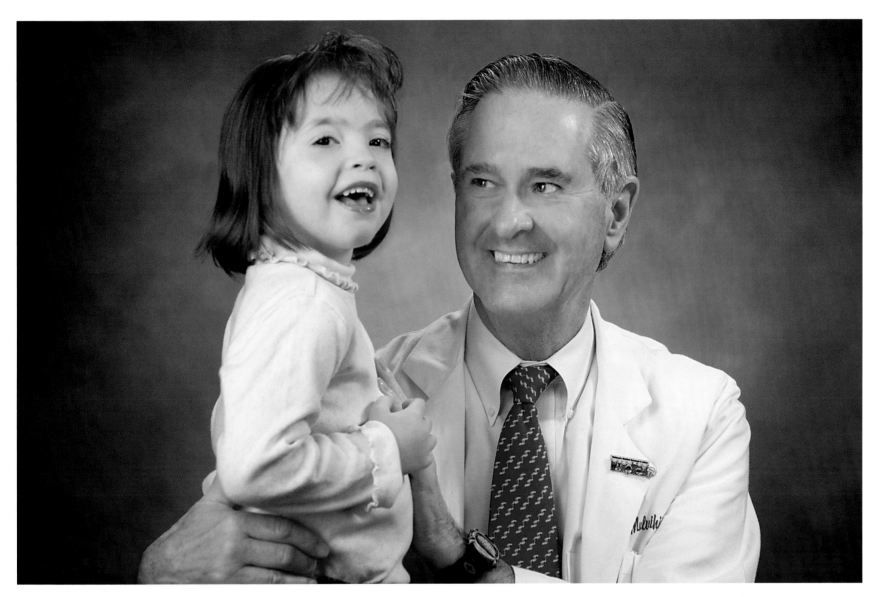

Dr. John Mulvihill has directed medical genetics at the OUHSC since 1998. He came to Oklahoma after earning an international reputation in the genetics of human cancer. *Courtesy Taylor Made Photography.*

region that did not have a comprehensive cancer treatment and research center.

Boren called upon the state legislature to use money from Oklahoma's share of the settlement of a multistate lawsuit against tobacco companies to help fund the cancer treatment center. Boren actively pursued private monies to match federal and state commitments. Boren and OU completed a Reach for Excellence campaign in 2000, raising more than $508 million.

"State Research Sees Enlightened Age" was the headline in a newspaper story in October, 2000, outlining the growth of research on the Oklahoma Health Center campus. Researcher Anne Pereira at the OUHSC was featured in the article as one of hundreds of scientists at OHC "who are part of a cultural change that is reorienting research nationwide." Technology transfer, born in the Silicon Valley in California decades before, was evident in Oklahoma.

Grants of more than $20 million in 2000 from NIH drew Oklahoma closer to the national average in biomedical research funding for state laboratories. Money from grants to OUHSC and OMRF funded a center devoted to examining how infectious organisms cause disease and provided research funds for scientists investigating autoimmune diseases, cancer, and cardiovascular diseases.

In the latest of many name changes, the old University, Children's, and Presbyterian hospitals became the "OU Medical Center" in 2001. It was a brilliant marketing idea. For several years, the hospitals were known as University Health Partners, but that name did not give citizens the full story of the amazing progress being made in the OU College of Medicine, the OUHSC, the teaching hospitals, and Presbyterian Hospital.

At the same time, University Physicians, the growing group of doctors practicing primarily in the hospitals, became OU Physicians. The group was preparing to move the practices of 156 of its 400 doctors to a 178,000-square-foot medical office building being built on the OUHSC campus. OU Physicians had become the largest multispeciality-speciality group in the state and included doctors who care for adult and pediatric patients across Oklahoma. The physicians were also on the faculty of the OU College of Medicine.

"It was finally the right branding," said Hershel Lamirand, president of the Oklahoma Health Center Foundation. "All at once, citizens identified the medical center and the medical school with OU's excellence." OU President Boren said, "Adding OU's name to the medical center completes nearly a century of OU's commitment to medical care at that location. This is a huge concentration of medical talent in one place and the use of the university's name highlights that for us."

In the early part of the new century, Stanton L. Young saw what he had been dreaming of for decades—the migration of top-flight medical researchers to Oklahoma. It was evident that doctors and scientists from prestigious medical centers across the nation were relocating at the Oklahoma Health Center for many reasons. A growing research park attracted private companies to commercialize biomedical discoveries. Endowed chairs funded by groups such as the Children's Medical Research Institute and the Presbyterian Health Foundation allowed the hiring of sought-after researchers and physicians. For example, the Donald W. Reynolds Foundation established chairs in geriatrics.

Young said, "What we have seen has been the attraction of researchers to the state that ultimately will improve patient care for our citizens. It's the best of both worlds. We gain incredible jobs and our citizens will have access the latest in medical technology and treatment. Research is the future of the Oklahoma Health Center."

Dr. Joseph Ferretti echoed Young's perspective. Ferretti said, "Advances in biomedical research not only ensures that Oklahomans will have better medical care, but it translates into high-technology jobs which will boost Oklahoma's economy." Randy Goldsmith, former president of the Oklahoma Technology Commercialization Center, said, "So what is the message here? The starting gun has been fired on what is the equivalent of the great Oklahoma land run in science and technology."

An example of the new world of private companies interacting with OHC researchers was ProteomTech, Inc., in 2001. The company planned to grow proteins found in the human body to be marketed to scientists worldwide for up to $1 million per gram. "The proteins will be used to create ways to fight illnesses, even some that may now be untreatable," said Henry Lin, chief scientific officer of the company. The proteins were to be grown in bacteria in China and then shipped to the company's headquarters in Oklahoma City. The idea worked.

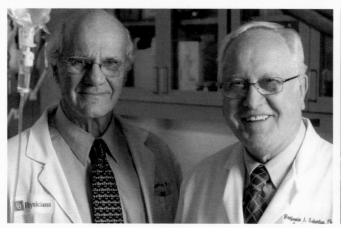 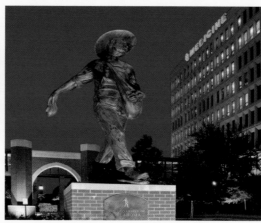 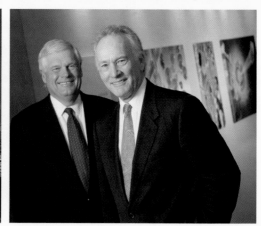

Chapter Eight

Oklahoma's Next Oilfield

Oklahoma always will be known as the place of some of the greatest oil discoveries on the planet. However, many observers believe the economic impact of the Oklahoma Health Center will give black gold a race for its money. A report on the national economy published by the Progressive Policy Institute compared all 50 states and ranked Oklahoma seventh in economic dynamism, a reflection of state, university, and private efforts to develop the Oklahoma Health Center.

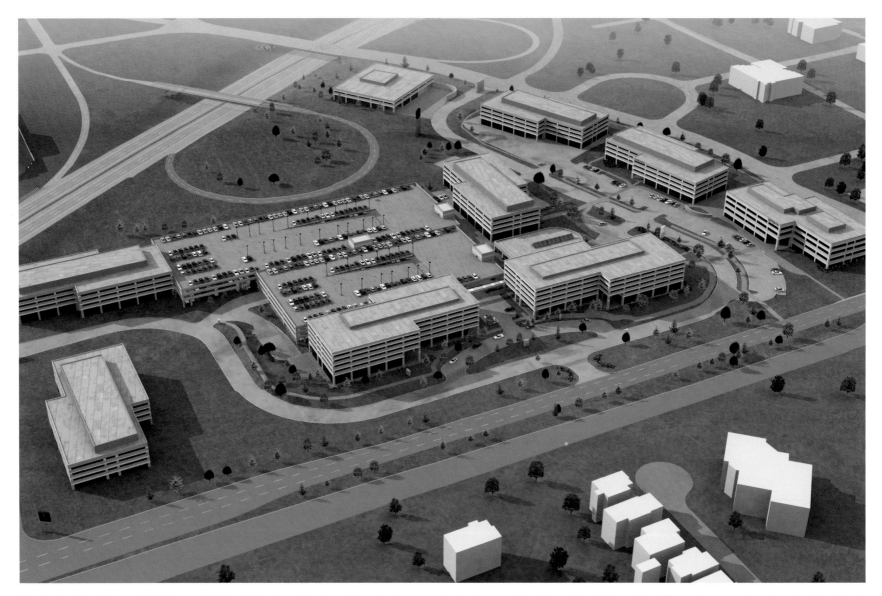

The Presbyterian Research Park is west of Lincoln Boulevard and contains private companies that are reaching into medical future with cutting-edge research and application of past research. *Courtesy Presbyterian Health Foundation.*

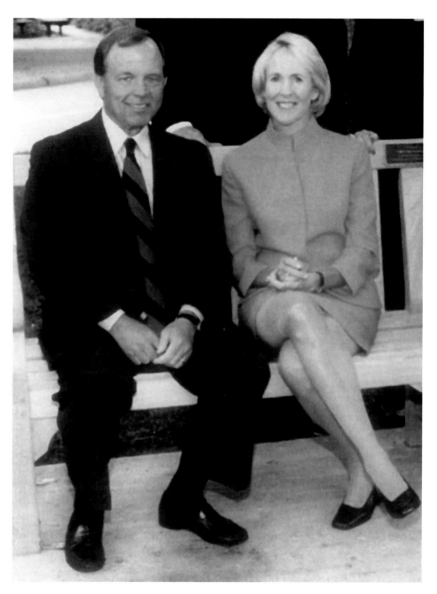

Jim and Christy Everest have been strong supporters of excellence at the Oklahoma Health Center. As chairman of the Oklahoma Health Center Foundation board, Jim led policymakers in assuring sound growth of the institutions on the OHC campus. *Courtesy Oklahoma Publishing Company.*

*I*n 2002, after the first three buildings in the PHF Research Park were fully leased, project architect Bud Miles gave reporters an explanation of two new buildings on the campus— a new $16 million, 125,000-square-foot research building and a $3 million commercial building. The new commercial building, unlike the multi-story structures previously built in the research park, was intended to attract retail stores and service companies to serve the park's growing research and technical work force.

Economic statistics proved the amazing success story. By 2002, more than 10,000 high-paying technology jobs had been created in Oklahoma—jobs that paid between $50,000 and $100,000 annually. Rudy Alvarado, chairman of Advancia Corp., said, "The state is creating sustainable, high-salaried jobs and wealth not seen since the days of the oil boom."

Alvarado pointed to reports that 12,500 Oklahomans were employed at institutions located at the Oklahoma Health Center, with an annual payroll of more than half a billion dollars. The base of medical research had expanded to cover biotechnology, bioinformatics, proteomics, and nanotechnology. Several groups

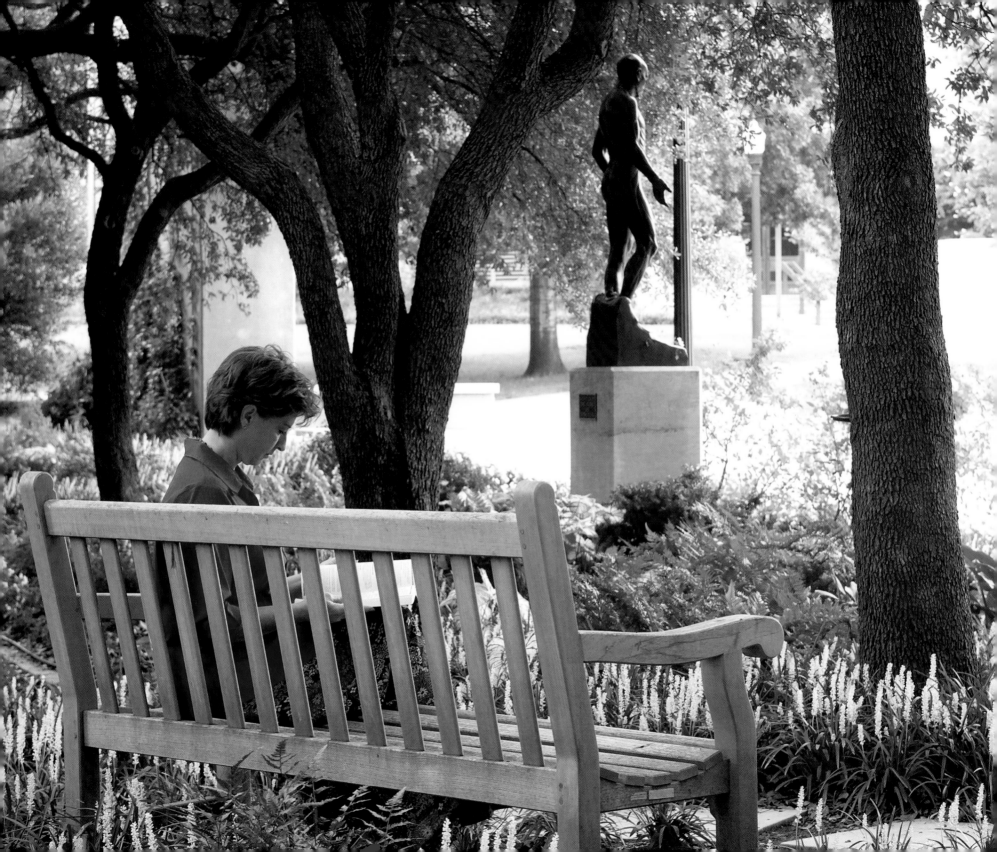

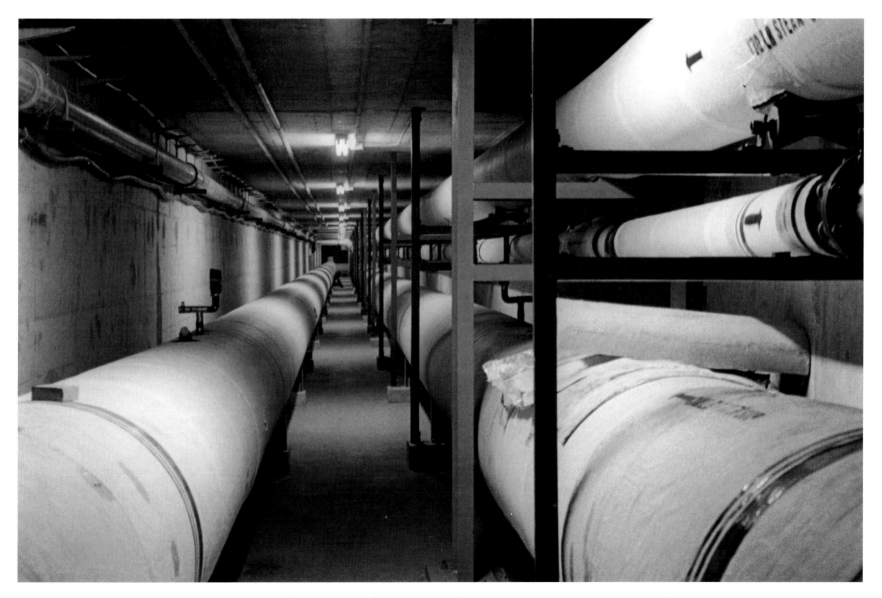

Beneath the buildings and parking lots that make up the Oklahoma Health Center are miles of steam lines, water and sewage pipes, and utilities.
Courtesy *Robert M. Bird Health Sciences Library.*

(Facing page) A calm and shady setting for students and faculty is provided by a grove of live oak trees in a garden on the OUHSC campus. In the garden is the Anatomical Donor Memorial by OU artists-in-residence Paul Moore and Veida Blick. The statue was given by the OU College of Medicine Class of 2001 to honor those who donate their bodies to science. *Courtesy OU College of Medicine.*

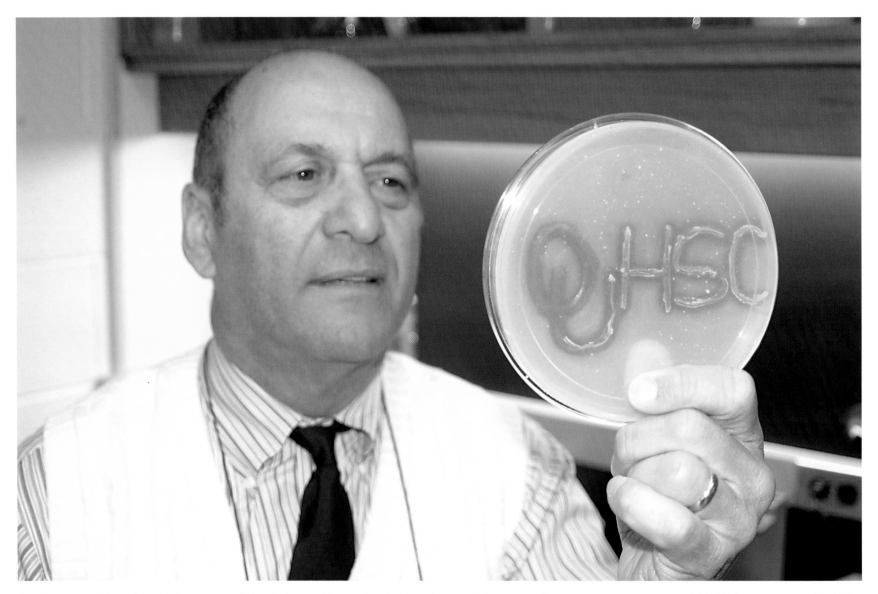

Dr. John Iandolo, Chair of the OU Department of Microbiology and Immunology, holds a plate on which voracious E.coli-eating microbe spell out OUHSC. Scientists at the OUHSC are conducting many projects to find out more about killer microbes that affect humans and animals worldwide. *Courtesy OU College of Medicine.*

The State Chamber

The Oklahoma Health Center is a key hub of business in the center of our state. With more than 30 health and research institutions, three major hospitals, and the Health Sciences Center, OHC is critical to Oklahoma's success. The number of employees and the economic impact is huge.

But more than economic impact is the tremendous positive force OHC entities provide on the health and well being of our citizens. The institutions are focused on improving the health, and health care, of our communities. The social missions of teaching, research, high-tech services, innovation in care, and the care of the indigent cannot be overstated.

OHC has placed Oklahoma on the map for innovative research and the contributions resulting from that research have been recognized around the world. We are blessed to have the leadership and commitment at the Oklahoma Health Center.

Dick Rush, President and CEO
The State Chamber of Oklahoma

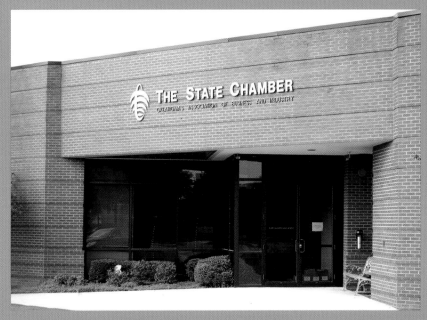

The State Chamber of Oklahoma's headquarters is on the Oklahoma Health Center campus. *Courtesy Eric Dabney.*

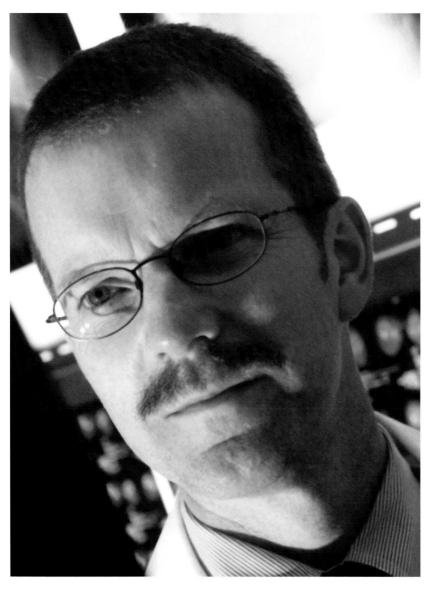

Dr. David Teague, chair of the OU Department of Orthopedic Surgery and Rehabilitation.
Courtesy University of Oklahoma.

were feverishly working to find the cause of or cure for many diseases. Alvarado said, "This growth is the result of more than good fortune. Rather, it is the result of clear, strategic thinking, planning, and investment."

In addition to building concrete and steel structures to house the Oklahoma Health Center's blossoming growth, a 2002 dedication of new central campus gardens of the OUHSC gave "a whole new face" to the area. The gardens, part of the OU beautification program led by OU First Lady Molly Boren, tied together for the first time the many buildings of the OUHSC. It was one of the largest landscaping projects in the history of the state with thousands of trees and shrubs, blooming flowers, fountains, sculpture, benches, and brick sidewalks. The $6.25 million beautification project was endowed with private donations.

The focal point of the project is the Stanton L. Young Walk, honoring the Oklahoma businessman, civic leader, and humanitarian. The walk replaced a divided road with a seven-tiered garden featuring traditional OU gates at each end.

Anchoring the west entrance of the walk in the Seed Sower sculpture by OU artist-in-residence Paul Moore. The Presbyterian Health Foundation Trustees Fountain is named to honor OU's largest private donor for its dedication and generosity. On the east end of the walk, the Thelma Gaylord Memorial Clock Tower and Gateway Arch greet visitors with traditional OU songs in chimes at each quarter hour. The gift honors the memory of Oklahoma City civic leader Thelma Gaylord, wife of publisher Edward L. Gaylord. Other gardens were made possible by gifts of George and Nancy Records, OG&E Electric Services, the Oklahoma Health Center Foundation, the College of Medicine Class of 2001, and physicians who donated to a special campaign.

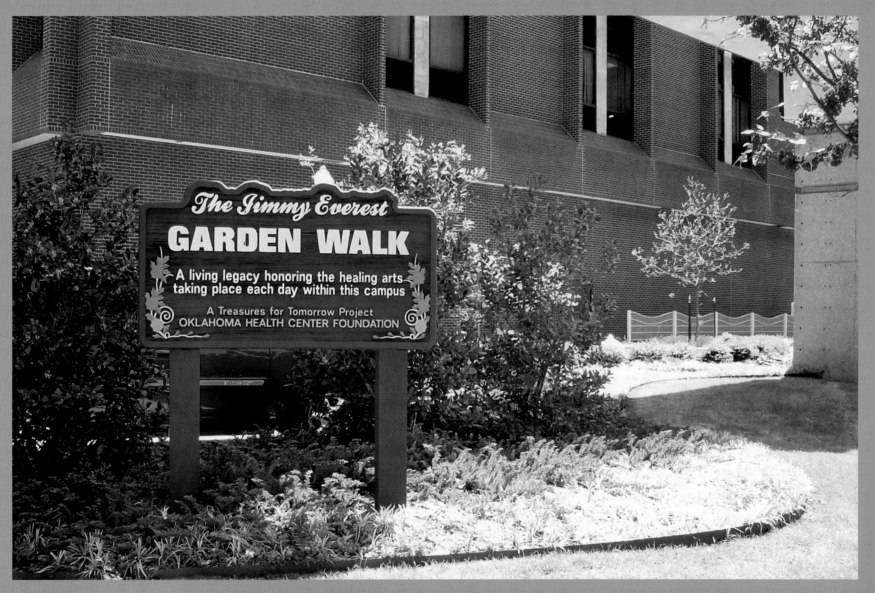

A 2001 project of Treasures for Tomorrow and the Oklahoma Health Center Foundation was the Jimmy Everest Garden Walk, a park-like setting that provides guests with a supportive, nurturing environment on the OHC campus. *Courtesy Oklahoma Health Center Foundation.*

Treasures for Tomorrow

In 2000, civic leader Sue Ann Hyde led an effort to establish an annual event to pay tribute to citizens whose lives served as models in the community and raise money for beautification and major art expressions on the OHC campus. Modeled after a similar program in Santa Fe, New Mexico, Treasures for Tomorrow honors prominent members of the community. Event proceeds and project donors have funded the Live Oak Grove, the Jimmy Everest Garden Walk, and the Beacon of Hope. Dean A. McGee Eye Institute is matching funds raised through the Treasures program to build a multi-dimensional glass sculpture titled "New Horizon," to be placed on the DMEI grounds. The project's completion date is 2010.

Treasures for Tomorrow Honorees

2000
Rick Bayless
Greg Burns
Robert and Harriette Orbach
Robert S. Kerr, Jr.
Stanton L. Young

2001
Marion Briscoe Devore
Gene Rainbolt
Jim and Beth Tolbert
Jim Vallion

2002
Ann Simmons Alspaugh
Dr. Michael Anderson
Dr. Edward Brandt
Dan Little
Chris Lower
Dick and Jeannette Sias

2003
Jean Gumerson
Karen Luke
Leonard McMurry
Dr. Paul Sharp

2004
Ray and Lou Ackerman
Mex Frates
Rabbi A. David Packman
Bert Seabourn

2005
Josephine Freede
James and Madalynne Norick
Drs. Ron Gilcher and Don Rhinehart
Hal Smith

2006
Avis Scaramucci
Ray and Pat Potts
Max Weitzenhoffer
George and Donna Nigh

2007
Ronald J. Norick
Nick Demos and Paula Stover
Larry and Polly Nichols
John W. Rex

2008
Joel Levine
Dr. Joseph J. and Mrs. Martha Ferretti
Bob Burke
Burns Hargis
Michael Turpen

2009
Ben Harjo
Don Karchmer
Lee Allan Smith
J. Blake Wade
Tom and Judy Love

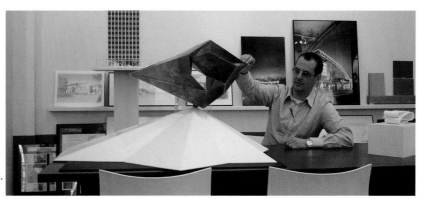

The multi-dimensional glass sculpture planned for the grounds of the Dean A. McGee Eye Institute is the project of designers Shan Shan Sheng and Mark Dziewulski, shown with a working model of the sculpture. Proceeds from recent Treasures of Tomorrow banquets, sponsored by the Oklahoma Health Center Foundation, and a gift from Dr. David Parke, Sr., will make possible the sculpture that will be ten feet tall and 18 feet wide and will be erected in front of the latest addition to the Dean A. McGee Eye Institute. *Courtesy Michael Joseph.*

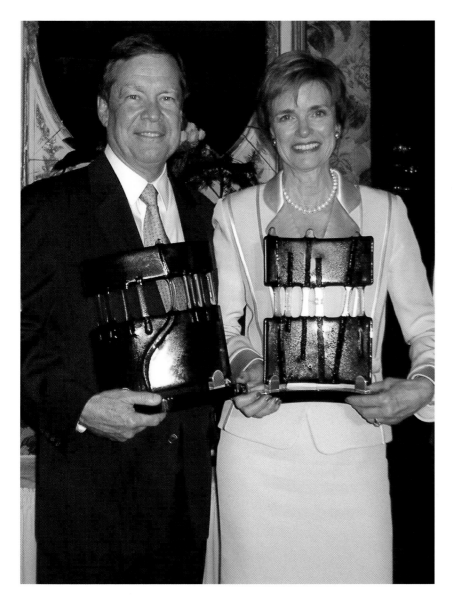

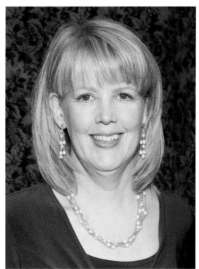

In 2007, Devon Energy Corporation co-founder Larry Nichols, left, and his wife, Polly, were honored as Treasures for Tomorrow by the Oklahoma Health Center Foundation. Money raised from the annual event funds beautification projects on the OHC campus. *Courtesy Oklahoma Health Center Foundation.*

Mary Kay Audd, staff assistant and special events coordinator for the Oklahoma Health Center Foundation.

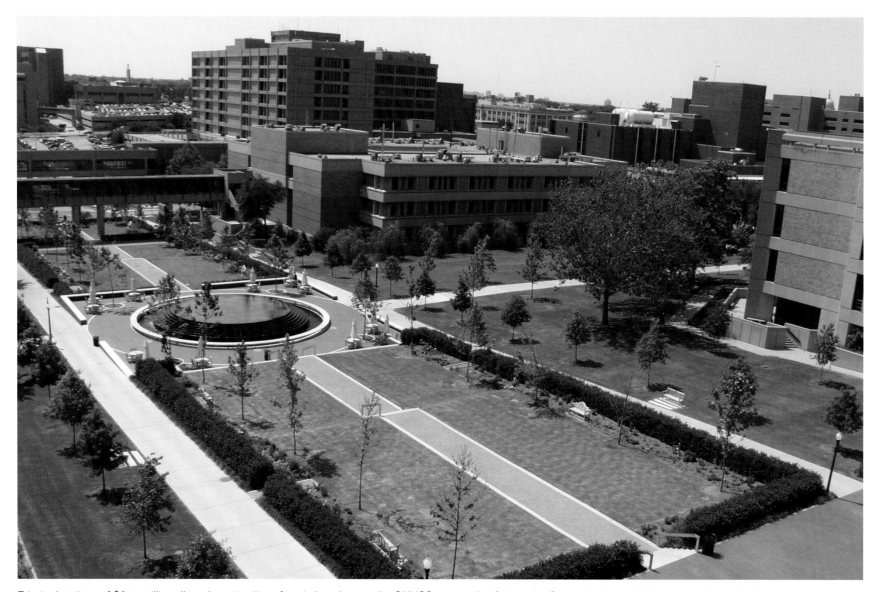

Private donations of $6.25 million allowed construction of central gardens on the OUHSC campus that feature the Stanton L. Young Walk, a pedestrian mall with seven tiered gardens. *Courtesy University of Oklahoma.*

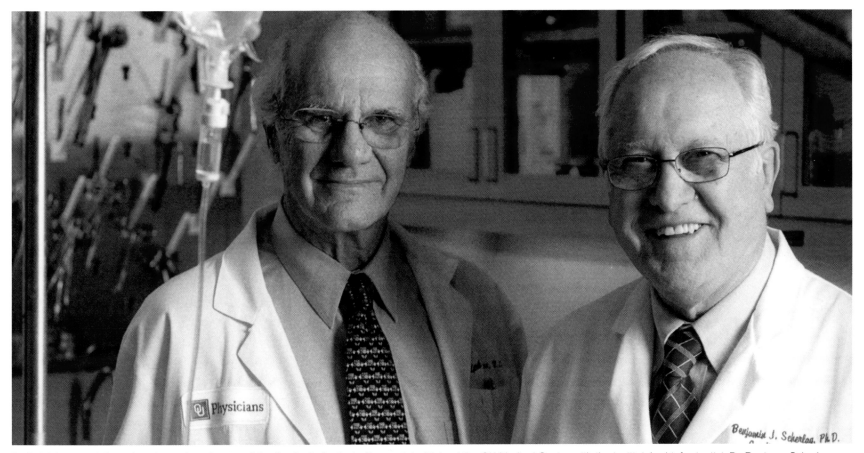

Dr. Ralph Lazzara, left, co-founder and co-director of the Cardia Arrthythmia Research Institute at the OU Medical Center with the institute's chief scientist, Dr. Benjamn Scherlag. *Courtesy OUCollege of Medicine.*

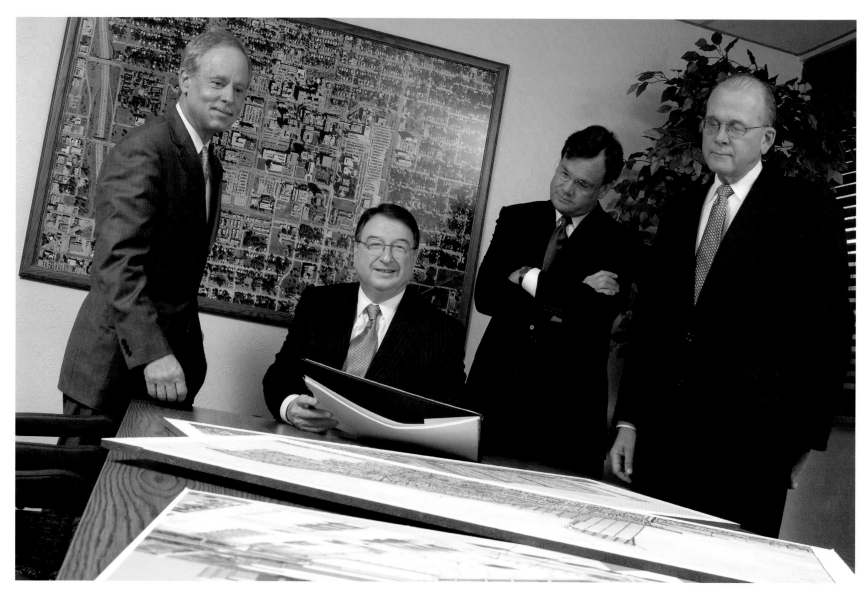

Planning for the future of the Oklahoma Health Center campus are, left to right, Dean Gandy, executive director of the University Hospitals Authority and Trust; Dr. M. Dewayne Andrews, executive dean of the OU College of Medicine; Authority and Trust Chairman Mike Samis; and Jerry Meier, then CEO of the OU Medical Center. *Courtesy OU College of Medicine.*

Dr. J. Donald Capra, president and scientific director of the Oklahoma Medical Research Foundation, bragged on the accomplishments of partners in the Oklahoma Health Center in a "Point of View" article in *The Daily Oklahoman* in December, 2002. He emphasized that the future of the state's economy lies with biotechnology, not solely oil and agriculture that fueled the state for its first century. Dr. Capra said, "Fortunately, the seeds for reshaping the entrepreneurial landscape have already been planted, and their fruits are evident in the biotechnology ventures rapidly springing up across the state."

Dr. Capra cited statistics of $60 million in National Institutes of Health grants secured for his organization and OUHSC researchers for the year. He said, "Combine this total with the estimated $40 million-plus these entities also received in other grant funding, and biomedical research and biotechnology added more than $100 million in out-of-state dollars to Oklahoma's economy."

"But, that is only the beginning," Dr. Capra wrote. He said, "In the world of biotechnology, patents represent a revenue source that can dwarf grant monies. When scientists make a discovery, a patent ensures that the scientist (or their employer) own the rights to the discovery. If another entity—say a pharmaceutical company— wants access to the discovery, that entity will have to pay the inventor."

OMRF owns more than 500 domestic and international patents. Dr. Capra said, "If even one of those patented discoveries results in the development of a new drug, OMRF, and the Oklahoma economy, could reap tens of millions of dollars." OMRF is only one of dozens of in-state biomedical research and biotechnology organizations that could provide a huge boost to the state's economy in the future.

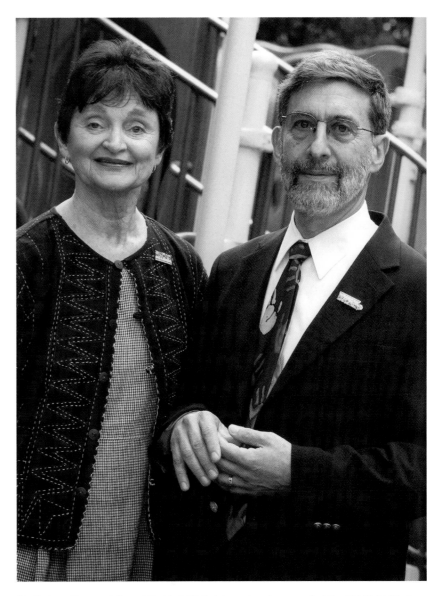

Dr. Barbara Bonner, left, and Dr. Mark Wolraich on the playground of the OU Child Study Center. Wolraich is director of the center that combines evaluation, training, treatment, and research, all designed to improve the lives of Oklahoma children with special needs, form autism and learning disabilities to abuse and neglect. *Courtesy OU college of Medicine.*

127

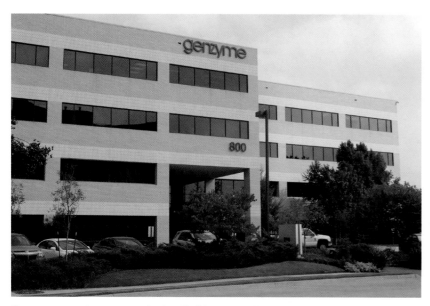

Genzyme occupies space in the 800 Building at the Presbyterian Health Foundation Research Park. *Courtesy Eric Dabney.*

British pharmaceutical giant AstraZeneca announced largescale human clinical trials to test Cerovive, a new drug to treat strokes. The drug had its roots at OMRF and the laboratory of scientist Robert Floyd. In the late 1980s, Floyd and a team of researchers discovered a compound that prevented and even reversed brain injury when given to animals a full hour after a stroke.

At OMRF, scientists Charles Esmon and Dr. Fletcher Taylor made important discoveries about the treatment of severe sepsis, a blood disease that kills an average of one person per minute in the world. Eli Lilly and Co. licensed the Oklahoma scientists' work and used it to develop Xigris, the first FDA-approved treatment for sepsis. In its first full year on the market, Xigris topped $100 million in sales.

Dr. William Canfield of OUHSC developed a compound for the treatment of Pompe disease, a rare and sometimes fatal muscular disease. The discovery resulted in Genzyme conducting clinical trials. OMRF official Larry Kennedy said, "As these Oklahoma-born products reach hospitals and pharmacies, royalties from their sales come back to the state. These revenues help create more high-quality, high-salary jobs for Oklahomans. And these new jobs, in turn, help us make further inroads against disease."

On January 1, 2003, Dr. Michael Anderson was named president and Carl Edwards was chosen chairman of the Presbyterian Health Foundation. Jean Gumerson became chairman and president emeritus. Anderson, a member of the foundation's board of directors since its inception, was chair of the grants committee which funds medical research and life science industry. He had served as senior minister of Oklahoma City's Westminster Presbyterian Church for 25 years. Edwards, a member of the foundation board since 1994, was co-managing partner of Price

(Facing page) Carl Edwards, left, chairman of the Presbyterian Health Foundation board and PHF President Dr. Michael Anderson. *Courtesy John Jernigan.*

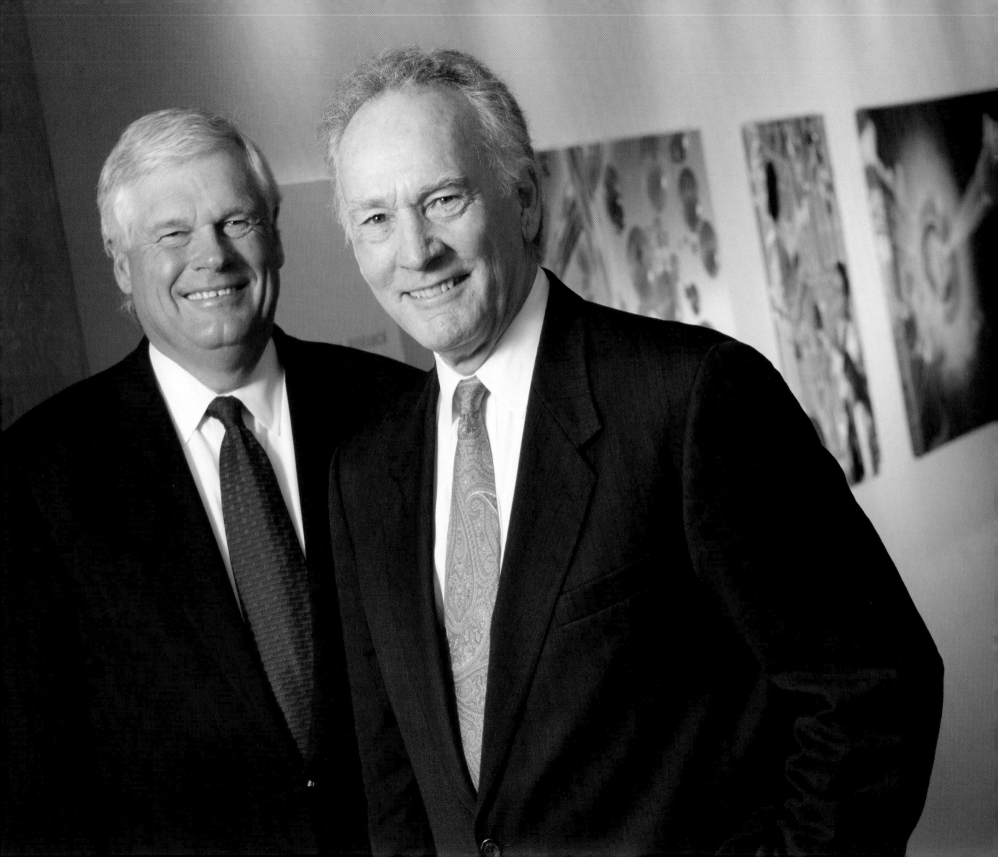

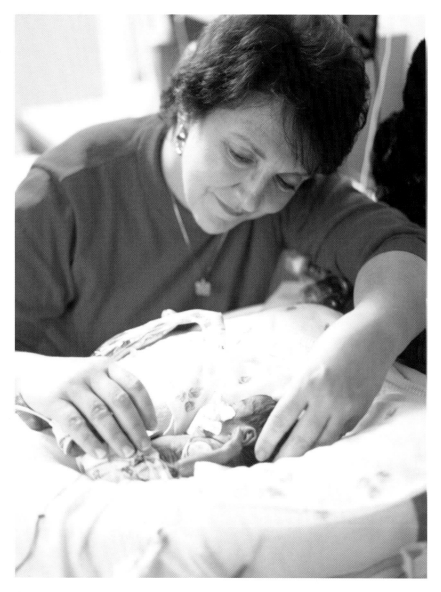

Dr. Marilyn Escobedo with a tiny patient in the neonatal intensive care unit of Children's Hospital at OU Medical Center. Dr. Escobedo holds the Children's Medical Research Institute-Reba McEntire Chair in Neonatology and is chair of the Neonatal-Perinatal Section in the OU Department of Pediatrics. *Courtesy Children's Medical Research Foundation.*

Edwards & Company of Oklahoma City, a commercial real estate service company. Edwards was also chairman of the Oklahoma Health Center Foundation.

One of the first grants awarded under Dr. Anderson's administration was a $2 million grant to help propel Oklahoma researchers into the forefront of genetics study. In late January, 2003, the foundation announced the grant to help OUHSC and OMRF researchers investigate genes, an area of research revolutionizing the fields of diagnostics, therapeutics, and drug discovery. More than 30 OUHSC researchers were focusing on genetics and almost a third of the OMRF grant money was dedicated to genetic research.

PHF also announced a commitment to provide $5 million to aid in the building of the second phase of the Stanton L. Young Biological Research Center on the OUHSC campus. The center is dedicated to genetics and cancer research.

In May, 2003, a Finland-based biotech company announced it would establish its American headquarters in Oklahoma City at the Oklahoma Health Center. Inion, Inc., maker of biodegradable materials used in bone regeneration, chose office space at the PHF Research Park. The company made Inion Hexalon, a colored screw used to repair bone and joint injuries. Inion chose Oklahoma City because of the progressive leadership of the PHF Research Park, the OUHSC, and the fact that a national survey showed Oklahoma City as one of the most affordable cities in the nation, with the cost of living at eight percent below the national average.

Attracting Inion showed that the park could lure more than just local entrepreneurs. PHF Chairman Carl Edwards said, "This shows we look good to companies around the world." Larry Kennedy, vice president of technological transfer for OMRF told a reporter, "It's one thing to try to fill it up with companies that are grown organically here, but it's even more successful if you can bring in established companies from outside the area because you're bringing in new money and new people."

The rich environment brought about the growth of such companies as Inoveon Corp, which was using technology developed at the OUHSC to detect and monitor eye disease. Dr. William Hagstrom the company's chairman said, "We are flourishing in part because of the nurturing infrastructure. We have access to technology, space, capital, and talent." Hagstrom was the former chairman of UroCor. He called Oklahoma City's growth in the bio-tech world "phenomenal."

By December, 2003, *The Daily Oklahoman* said biotechnology had emerged as "the engine that will fuel the state's economic growth for decades," or at least "has had a major effect on Oklahoma." Business writer Jim Stafford noted that technology stories had dominated the year's business headlines including the Oklahoma Nanotechnology Initiative passed by the Oklahoma legislature.

In 2004, Governor Brad Henry's EDGE committee began putting forth ideas to transform Oklahoma into the "research capital of the Plains." EDGE—Economic Development Generating Excellence—committee members brainstormed up to a $1 billion endowment to turn Oklahoma into a research mecca. Many of the ideas that surfaced dealt with selling state assets. Burns Hargis, chairman of the Greater Oklahoma City Chamber of Commerce, suggested state office buildings be sold on a "lease-back" basis to help build an endowment to earn large amounts of interest for investment in scientists and laboratory space.

John Frick, general partner of Chisholm Capital Partners, a

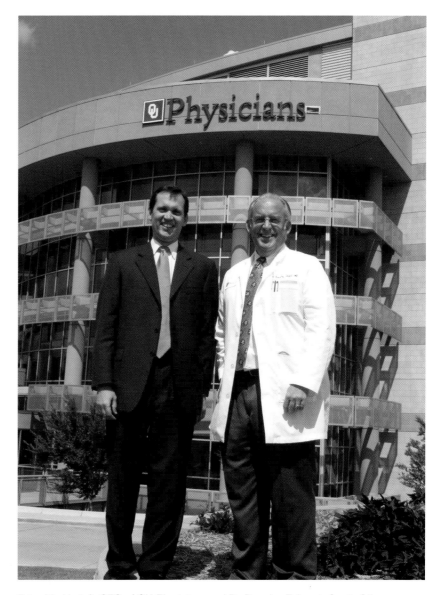

Brian Maddy, left, CEO of OU Physicians and Dr. Douglas Folger in front of the new OU Physicians Building in 2003. *Courtesy OU College of Medicine.*

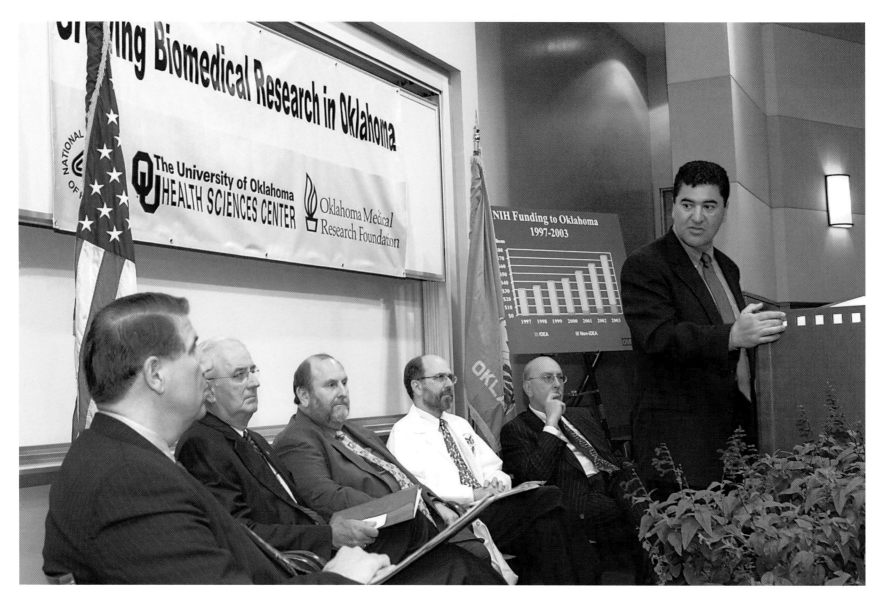

Dr. Elias Zerhouni, at the podium, director of the National Institutes of Health, announced a $17.95 million grant in June, 2004, to build Oklahoma's capacity to carry out biomedical research by supporting promising young faculty investigators. It was the largest grant ever awarded to an Oklahoma institution. Left to right, Congressman Ernest Istook, Jr., OUHSC Provost Dr. Joseph Ferretti, Dr. Frank Waxman, Dr. John Harley, and Dr. Donald Capra, president of the Oklahoma Medical Research Foundation. *Courtesy OU College of Medicine.*

venture capital company active in funding start-up companies, predicted the EDGE endowment could generate $50 million a year to seed matching research grants to double the amount of federal money coming to the state. Greg Main, president of i2E, said, "The Oklahoma Health Center provides a perfect blueprint for an endowment suggested by EDGE. The proximity of the research park to the nearby biotechnology research ongoing at the OUHSC and OMRF is the key."

The talk of funding research was against a backdrop of significant advances at the Oklahoma Health Center in combining research and commercialization of new discoveries. Dr. Paul Weigel was an excellent example. Weigel, chair of the biochemistry and molecular biology department at the OUHSC, co-founded Hyalose LLC, a company commercializing the technology he developed in the laboratory. Dr. Joseph Waner, director of the OUHSC office of technology development, estimated that more than 100 patents had been obtained by OU scientists in the previous six years. The year before, OU researchers won a record $41.1 million in research grants from the National Institutes of Health.

Michael Gilmore, vice president for research at OUHSC, identified the departments of microbiology, ophthalmology, and urology, as having made giant strides in acquiring additional NIH funding. In 2003, microbiology and ophthalmology were ranked in the Top 10 nationally in NIH grants, while urology was ranked No. 13.

OUHSC Senior Vice President and Provost, Dr. Joseph Ferretti, a microbiology professor, has brought substantial research funding to the OUHSC campus, primarily from the National Institutes of Health. Dr. Ferretti is an internationally recognized scientist who is known for his work in the area of infectious disease research,

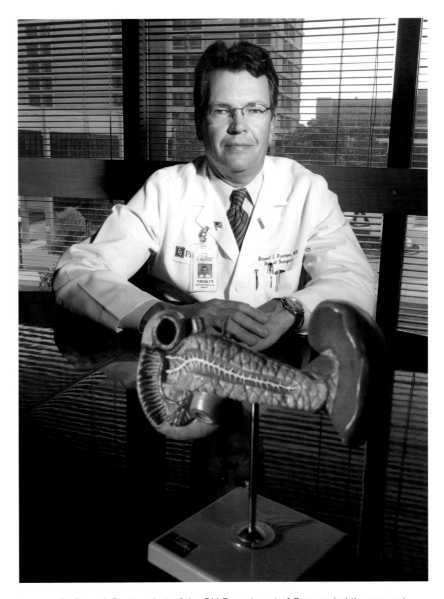

In 2004, Dr. Russell Postier, chair of the OU Department of Surgery, led the research effort to find a cure for pancreatic cancer that does not require surgery. Research at the OUHSC sought to understand the genetics of the dreaded disease. *Courtesy OU College of Medicine.*

Honoring Dr. Gilcher

In 2004, Dr. Ronald Gilcher, president, CEO, and chief medical officer of the Oklahoma Blood Institute was honored as "a visionary blood banker" by the Association of Donor Recruitment Professionals. The group named an annual award for Dr. Gilcher who was among the elite of blood bank directors in the nation. He inspired incredible growth of annual blood donor collections from 22,000 in 1979 to more than 200,000 in 2006 when he became OBI's medical director emeritus.

For many years, Dr. Gilcher led national efforts in blood center based public health programs. He pioneered cholesterol, prostate specific antigen (PSA), and cardiac disease marker testing for American donors. Similarly, for recipient safety, he was first to institute the HIV antigen test and single donor nucleic acid testing (NAT).

namely in the area of streptococcal infections and antibiotic resistance. Particularly noteworthy are his contributions to genetic engineering. He was the first scientist in Oklahoma to perform recombinant DNA experiments. He also established the microbial pathogen genome sequencing center.

Elsewhere on the OHC campus, OMRF researchers made news in 2004. Researchers John Harley and Judith James discovered certain proteins known as autoantibodies being present in the blood years before a person developed symptoms of lupus. Researchers believed these findings could prove crucial in treating approximately one million Americans suffering from lupus. OMRF scientist Robert Floyd's stroke treatment drug was entering large-scale human clinical trials and a pair of OMRF-based antibody drugs were being tested for use in cardiac bypass surgery and the treatment of heart attacks.

In July, 2004, Cytovance Biologics Inc., led by Dr. William Canfield, held a symbolic groundbreaking for a $16.8 million biopharmaceutical manufacturing plant at the PHF Research Park. It was the first pharmaceutical manufacturing facility in Oklahoma. The plant was approved by the Food and Drug Administration and was built to produce protein-based therapeutics and antibodies on a contract basis for biotechnology researchers and laboratories.

The Cytovance project was the result of several Oklahoma groups working with the Presbyterian Health Foundation. Before the manufacturing plant was announced, a full year of intense work had to be completed by BancFirst, the Oklahoma City Urban Renewal Authority, the Oklahoma City Redevelopment Authority, and Rural Enterprises of Oklahoma, a Durant-based, federally accredited community development financial institution.

Dr. J. Donald Capra, president of the Oklahoma Medical

Research Foundation, called upon state leaders to increase state funding in 2004 for OCAST. Funding had remained flat for several years for the agency, even though Capra called the center "the state's single most effective, efficient program for growing business."

During its first 17 years, OCAST had invested roughly $105 million in biotechnology, small businesses, manufacturing, and all kinds of homegrown entrepreneurial ventures. It was a major player in helping companies located in the Oklahoma Health Center.

Oklahoma's stature as a "heavyweight" in medical research received a huge boost in November, 2004, when the Dean McGee Eye Institute announced a $30 million expansion to its facilities on the OHC campus. The expansion was seen as proof of the institute's priority to bring the nation's finest research and clinical minds to Oklahoma City. In the previous decade, OU ophthalmology researchers at DMEI had jumped nationally from 64th to 8th in research support from the National Institutes of Health for eye care. By 2004, DMEI was home to 28 ophthalmologists staffing the adult and pediatric clinics and served 122,000 patients and performed 14,000 surgical procedures the previous year. Eighteen percent of the patient load was committed for Oklahomans who had no other access to specialized eye care.

In December, 2004, a wrecking ball slammed into the old research building at Northeast 13th Street and Phillips Avenue, clearing the way for a $110 million project to enhance health care for Oklahoma's children. The huge investment for the OU Children's Physicians Building was announced by Mike Samis, chair of the University Hospitals Authority and Trust. Samis reported by the time the new building was completed, the Trust's investment in capital improvements, medical education, research grants, and equipment would top $250 million.

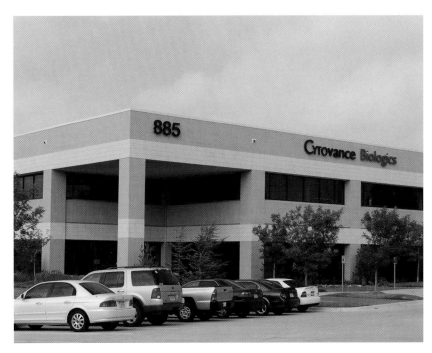

The Cytovance Biologics Building in the PHF Research Park was the first pharmaceutical manufacturing facility built in Oklahoma. *Courtesy Eric Dabney.*

Before the OU Children's Physicians Building, the single largest expenditure by the Trust was $22 million for construction of the OU Physicians Building for the faculty's adult practice. The new building was part of a master plan to consolidate the OU Medical Center from three to two physical structures.

The plan was for the former Presbyterian Hospital to focus on adult medical care, while Everett Tower would become a women's and children's hospital. The Trust's investment in the new facility was made possible by annual "rent" payments from Health Care Corporation of America.

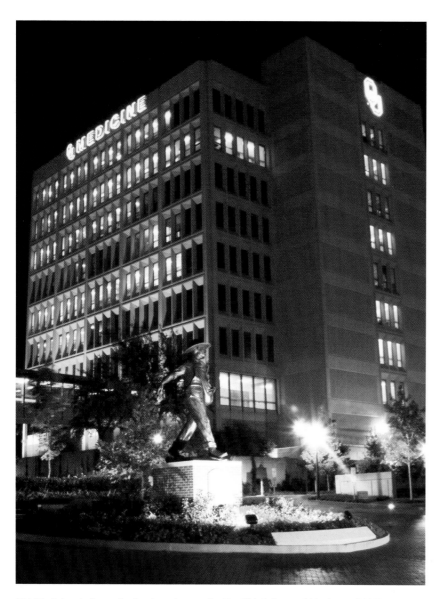

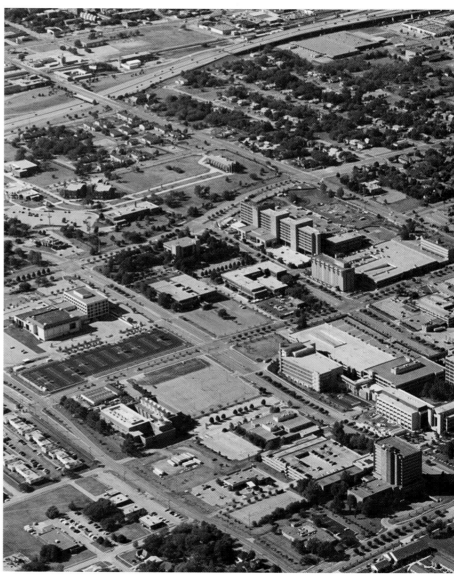

OU Medicine is the collective brand name for the OU College of Medicine, OU Physicians, University Hospitals Trust, and OU Medical Center, including The Children's Hospital. This sign is atop the Biomedical Sciences Building. *Courtesy OU College of Medicine.*

The rapid growth of the Oklahoma Health Center campus is shown in an aerial photograph in 2004. *Courtesy OU College of Medicine.*

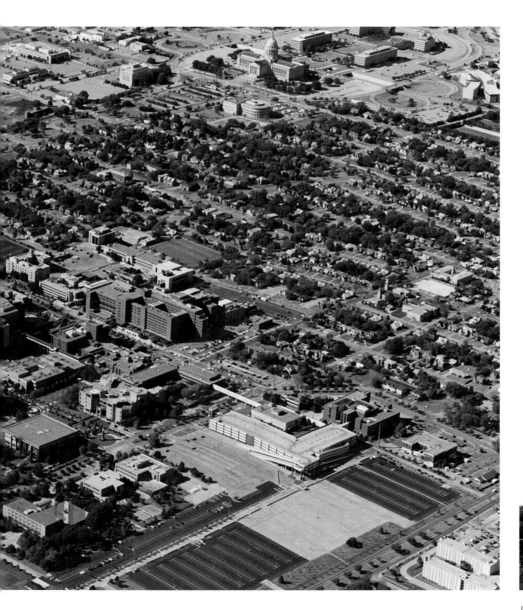

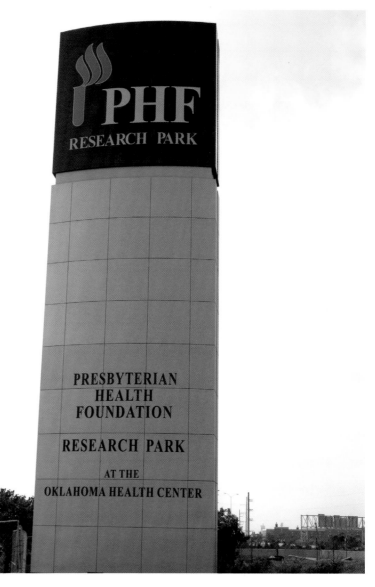

Unique signs along Interstate 235 announce the presence of the PHF Research Park. The signs alert citizens to the significant impact the research park is making on Oklahoma's economy. *Courtesy Eric Dabney.*

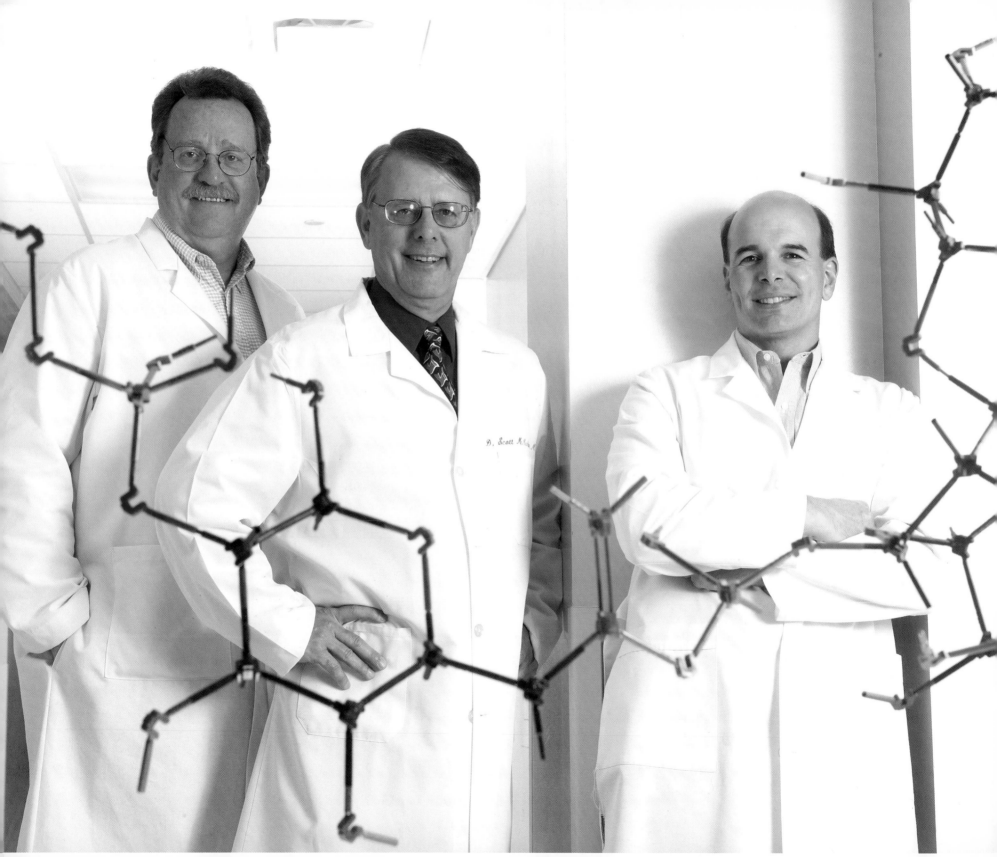

University of Oklahoma College of Medicine

The University of Oklahoma College of Medicine was established in 1900 as a medical department of the University of Oklahoma in Norman, initially offering two years of pre-clinical education. In 1911, the OU medical school merged with the Epworth College of Medicine in Oklahoma City to become a full four-year MD degree granting institution. By 1928, all of the pre-clinical and medical operations had been centralized in Oklahoma City at what would ultimately become the University of Oklahoma Health Sciences Center. The College is the largest component of the OU Health Sciences Center and is the focus of activities around which much of the Oklahoma Health Center has been developed over the past 45 years.

The College includes 4 basic sciences departments, 18 clinical departments, and 14 Centers of Excellence. The faculty practice, known as OU Physicians, is the largest medical group in Oklahoma, with almost 500 physicians representing every specialty and subspecialty of medicine. The College of Medicine faculty provides Oklahoma's largest concentration of biomedical research, annually bringing many millions of dollars of research grants to Oklahoma, contributing to the vitality of the Oklahoma Health Center and the economy of the city and state. The College has a branch clinical campus in Tulsa, established in 1974, which has been recently refocused as the School of Community Medicine, offering third and fourth year medical student education and residency training in 10 disciplines.

The College has over 600 medical students (162 new students enter each year), more than 600 residents and fellows in 52 specialty and subspecialty training programs, 150 physician assistant students, and 120 graduate students working on doctoral degrees in the biomedical sciences. The College has granted the MD degree to almost 9,000 individuals, more than half of whom ultimately practiced medicine in Oklahoma.

The College and its faculty have been responsible for developing the OU Cancer Institute, the Harold Hamm Oklahoma Diabetes Center, the OU Breast Institute, the Oklahoma Center for Neurosciences, the Heart Rhythm Research Institute, the Oklahoma Center on Aging, and the Center on Child Abuse and Neglect to name a few of its special centers. The OU Cancer Institute represents the largest single biomedical project ever undertaken in Oklahoma and will have tremendous impact on cancer research and cancer care throughout the state.

Where health care and the quality of life are concerned, the OU College of Medicine has played a critical role in Oklahoma's past and present, and it promises to have an even more important role in the future. The College is the major center for educating and training the future physician workforce for the state; it is the largest hub of biomedical research in Oklahoma; and the College's physicians provide health care to hundreds of thousands of Oklahomans each year and attract many individuals from outside Oklahoma because of some highly specialized areas of expertise and care. A vibrant medical school and successful academic medical center are critical to Oklahoma's continuing development and success. And they are the heart of the Oklahoma Health Center.

Dr. M. Dewayne Andrews
Vice President for Health Affairs
Executive Dean, College of Medicine

(Facing page)Three OU College of Medicine biochemists were leaders in the international effort in 2004 to study glycomics, the third leg of the race to understand the body's most basic mechanisms. Left to right, Dr. Richard Cummings, Dr. Paul Weigel, chair of the Department of Biochemistry and Molecular Biology, and Dr. Paul DeAngelis. *Courtesy OU College of Medicine.*

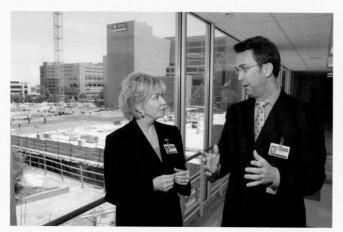
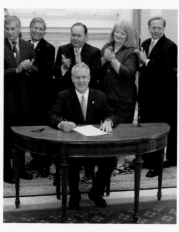
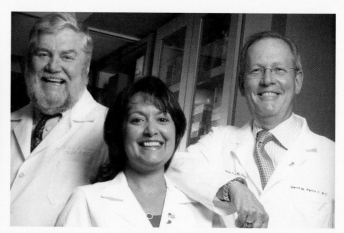

Chapter Nine

40 Years Old and Still Growing

The Oklahoma Health Center celebrated its 40th anniversary in 2005. It had made the leap from little more than an undefined concept to Oklahoma's premier resource for health care, research, medical education, and technology. OHC officials reflected on the growth.

Capital investment of $2.5 billion and nearly $2 billion in annual economic impact came from 12,500 jobs. Jim Killackey, staff writer for *The Daily Oklahoman*, wrote, "Now, the unique 300-acre complex between downtown Oklahoma City and the State Capitol…is a heavyweight conglomeration and concentration of 30 organizations ranging from the American Red Cross of Central Oklahoma to the Veterans Affairs Medical Center."

Killackey also wrote:

The Oklahoma Health Center has more than arrived in medical circles—there's nothing like it in the state, nothing quite like it in the United States. In so many ways, the campus is peerless and unequaled.

The world-class complex has become Oklahoma's shining epicenter for training tomorrow's medical professionals and finding solutions to the most complicated, most baffling diseases and ailments.

Patients come to the Oklahoma Health Center from all 77 counties for medical care provided by hundreds of physicians… Cutting-edge biotechnology companies have sprung up as if overnight in the research park. The campus has four hospitals, an adult daycare program, and the State Medical Examiner's Office.

Anywhere there's empty space on the bustling campus, plans are evolving to put something new on it.

OUHSC Provost Dr. Joseph Ferretti paid tribute to the more than 800 faculty members on campus. He said, "Our faculty is the bedrock of the campus…We have built a solid foundation for propelling us into the future."

A Bright Future for the PHF Research Park

Our mission, "to support medical research, and translational research leading to companies with innovative diagnostics and new therapeutics," bears evidence in the development of the PHF Research Park. The present configuration of the seven buildings of the Research Park is the home to 37 science based companies, 1500 employees, and an expansive near future growth for technicians, scientists and executives. One company alone projects a five year growth from 43 employees to 450. These innovative persons in highly skilled jobs offer Oklahoma a very strong technology base in the economic future. The average per capita income of Research Park personnel is three times the state average. New therapeutics and innovative diagnostics produced by these companies will enhance the health, save lives of Oklahomans and others worldwide.

An abridged list of our companies include Altheus (digestive diseases), Charlesson (therapeutics for eye disease), CoMentis (Alzheimer's disease treatment), Cytovance Biologics (cell banking and monoclonal antibody biopharmaceutical manufacturer), DNA Solutions (high quality DNA analytical technology contracts), Hyalose (unique recombinant technology focused on a polymer synthesis and creation of novel molecules), InterGenetics (genetic-based assessment test

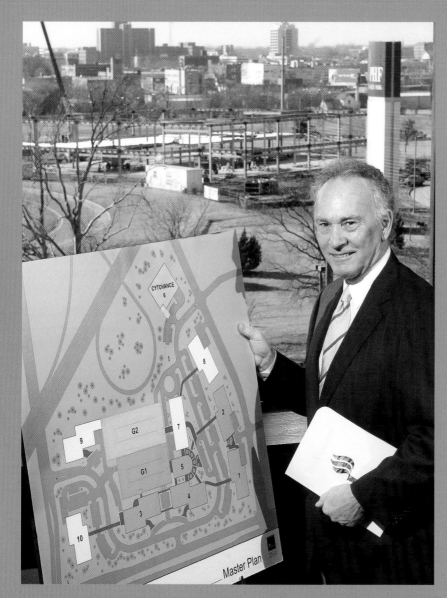

for various cancers) Lifetone (remote monitoring of life and health), OrthoCare (prosthetics research and development) Selexys (novel biopharmaceuticals for inflammatory and thrombotic diseases), Therametics (novel dermatological therapeutics).

Since, 1985 we have made more than $108 million in grants and developed a Research Park with 700,000 square feet of Class A wet lab and office space worth more than $120 million. We expect several of our biotech companies to be major companies in the near future affecting for good the whole State of Oklahoma.

We really are just starting. Some of the start-up companies are very small and young and some of them have extremely ambitious ideas. A few of them will work. The impact upon the economic future of Oklahoma is unlimited. In the coming decades, we will see a huge economic engine birthed on our campus.

Dr. Mike Anderson, President
Presbyterian Health Foundation

Presbyterian Health Foundation President Dr. Michael Anderson presents a master plan for development of the PHF Research Park. *Courtesy Oklahoma Publishing Company.*

Dr. Michael Anderson, president of the Presbyterian Health Foundation, used a newspaper guest editorial forum to tell success stories about biotech companies in 2005. Selexys Pharmaceuticals, one of the newest molecular technology companies, used science developed in the laboratories at OUHSC and OMRF for therapeutics to treat inflammatory and thrombotic diseases. Anderson said, "Selexys has a gigantic field to tackle," referring to inflammation's emergence as "the root of all illnesses."

Dr. Jordan Tang and his group used the name Zapaq for the discovery of a product to attack the plaque in brain cells. The product targets a group of enzymes central to Alzheimer's disease and gives great hope for a treatment to the debilitating disease.

Analytical Research Laboratories (ARL) and DNA Solutions (DNAS) also were major success stories at the PHF Research Park. ARL, one of the park's oldest tenants, was dedicated to providing analytical and quality control solutions for medicines compounded by pharmacists, from anti-aging creams to topical pain gels. ARL's services are used by regulatory agencies such as boards of pharmacy and pharmaceutical conventions.

DNAS was established in 2000 to provide genetic testing for humans, animals, and plants. The company provides human identification services for individuals to establish relationships for immigration, probate, child support, and criminal investigations. Also, DNAS uses cutting-edge technology to uniquely identify animals for prosecuting crimes involving animal theft and illegal hunting.

Dr. Tom Kupiec, president of ARL and DNAS, described joint ventures with scientists at OMRF to establish a genetic engineering database for various inflammatory conditions. "We are progressing by increasing research and development resources, improving facilities, developing a rapidly growing staff of multidisciplinary scientists, and conducting training for student interns."

While veteran researchers on the Oklahoma Health Center campus made discoveries, a future generation of leaders developed on the west side of the campus. In 2005, students at the Oklahoma School of Science and Mathematics again topped the state with their average ACT score and was among the best schools in the nation with its score on the college-entrance examination. Some years, OSSM ranked number one nationally on ACT scores. The 2005 class scored an average composite score of 31.3 out of a possible 36 points. The state's average score was 20.4.

In December, 2005, OMRF completed a fund-raising campaign that resulted in more than $100 million in gifts and pledges. Part of the money funded the $15 million Donald W. Reynolds Center for Genetic Research, a state-of-the-art facility housing about 25,000 mice used in a variety of experiments.

Not satisfied with the successful campaign, OMRF officials launched still another campaign, the Imagine Campaign, in hopes of raising another $100 million. OMRF president Dr. J. Donald Capra said, "Raising the $100 million by 2005 allowed us to imagine what we could do with another $100 million. Tomorrow, our labs could give birth to treatments for Alzheimer's disease, Lupus, or Lou Gehrig's disease. But for that to happen, we must have the tools to continue to recruit and retain top-caliber scientists."

OCAST selected Michael Carolina, an Oklahoma native with three decades of experience in the telecommunications industry, as its new executive director in 2005. The state's technology-based economic development agency won a small increase in state appropriations, although Carolina announced his goal was an increase in the agency's budget. He believed more money was needed to work for "sustainable economic development."

A 2005 poll conducted by Harris Interactive found Oklahomans were in favor of more medical and health research being conducted in the state. In fact, the poll indicated that 98 percent of the state's citizens questioned said it was important for Oklahoma to be a research leader.

The public's perception of Oklahoma's growth in medical research was helped by frequent media stories. In a five-week period in 2005, at least a half-dozen stories appeared in *The Daily Oklahoman* about private research companies located on the OHC campus. There was a feature story about Cytovance Biologics, Inc., opening its pharmaceutical production laboratory. "The start of the contract production business," PHF President Dr. Michael Anderson said, "represents a major milestone for both the company and the research park." Cytovance President William Fallon said the company would immediately begin offering cell culture, purification, and method development to biopharmaceutical drug developers. Another story traced the history of Dr. Jordan Tang and the race to find a cure for Alzheimer's disease.

Also in 2005, the ribbon was cut to officially open the $37.9 million expansion of the Stanton L. Young Biomedical Research Center. At the dedication, OU President Boren said the new project continues Oklahoma's pioneering spirit, "In the early days, our forefathers transformed the land. We could say that today our scientists are conquering new frontiers, coming with new discoveries and advancing knowledge. Phase II provides them with the tools they need to continue this mission."

The ceremony was used to announce two large grants from the National Institutes of Health. One grant, a renewal of an earlier

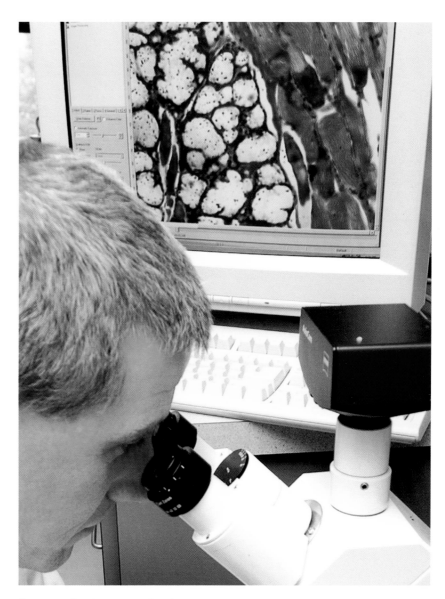

Dr. James Chodosh uses a digital microscope to look at a lacrimal gland from a primate eye at the Dean A. McGee Eye Institute. The research is part of the ongoing effort to improve eye care. *Courtesy Oklahoma Publishing Company.*

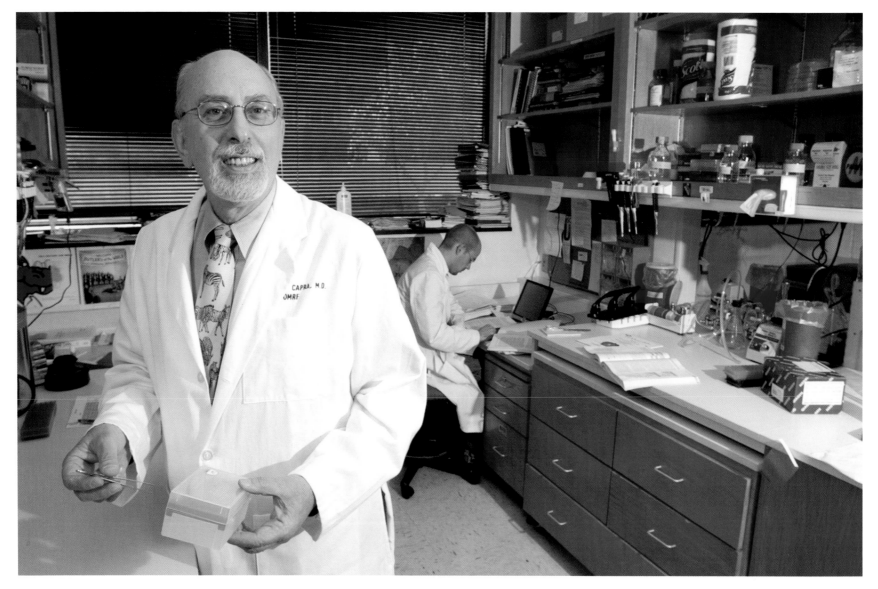

Dr. J. Donald Capra, past president of the Oklahoma Medical Research Foundation, in one of the foundation's research labs as graduate student Andy Duty works in the background. *Courtesy Oklahoma Publishing Company.*

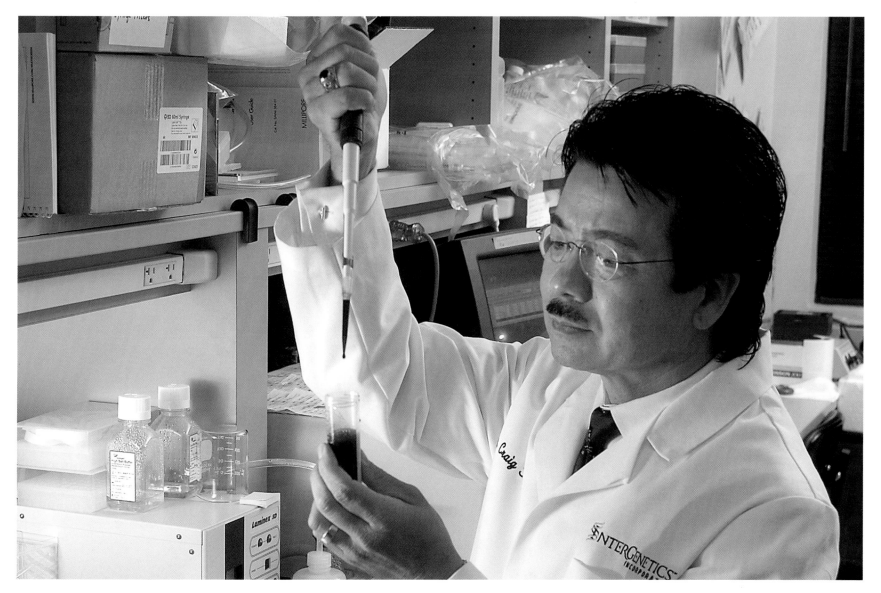

Craig Shimasaki works in the lab at InterGenetics, Inc., at the Presbyterian Health Foundation Research Park in 2005. *Courtesy Oklahoma Publishing Company.*

AH-CHOO

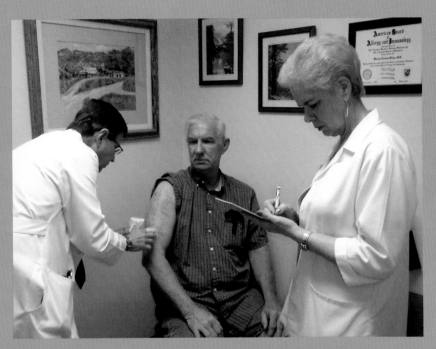

A major task for physicians and support personnel at the Oklahoma Allergy and Asthma Clinic is testing patients for allergic reactions. The clinic was founded in 1925 and is one of the largest and most respected diagnostic, treatment, and research centers of its kind. *Courtesy Oklahoma Allergy and Asthma Clinic.*

The Oklahoma Allergy and Asthma Clinic moved to the Oklahoma Health Center campus in 1980. The Clinic had its origins as the Balyeat Hay Fever and Asthma Clinic founded by Dr. Ray M. Balyeat in 1925. Upon his retirement, the name was changed to the Oklahoma Allergy Clinic. In 1995 its current title was updated to the Oklahoma Allergy and Asthma Clinic reflecting the overall scope of practice of the clinic.

It is one of the oldest and largest continuous practices of allergic diseases in the United States. Initially begun by four allergists, it has grown to a staff of eight Board Certified allergists and clinical immunologists as well as Board Certified pediatricians and internists and a Board Certified advanced practice nurse in allergy and asthma.

All physicians are either clinical faculty members of the Department of Internal Medicine or Department of Pediatrics in the University of Oklahoma College of Medicine. Teaching of medical students and graduate physicians has been one of the primary missions of the clinic. Patient care and clinical research round out the clinic's three missions. Diverse allergic and hypersensitivity problems are seen and treated, with an emphasis on respiratory disease.

Over the years, patients from not only the Southwest region of the United States have come to the Oklahoma Allergy and Asthma Clinic for evaluation and treatment but also virtually every state in America and numerous foreign countries. There are approximately 12,000 annual patient visits and 100,000 patient contacts.

Dr. John Bozalis

effort, went to the Department of Microbiology and Immunology to find answers to questions about the biological mechanisms of disease caused by infectious organisms. The second award, the largest ever received by OU from the National Cancer Institute, made funds available to help cancer prevention research.

Under the leadership of Senior Vice President and Provost Dr. Joseph Ferretti, the OUHSC began implementation of an aggressive five-year plan to significantly increase total biomedical research funding on the campus. The plan followed a five-year doubling of NIH grants to OUHSC. It centered on research development in the areas of cancer, diabetes and metabolic disease, neuroscience/vision, and infectious/immune system diseases.

The new strategic initiative for cancer research was a follow-up to the 2004 passage of an increased tobacco tax earmarked, in part, to secure a bond issue to build and provide equipment for the OU Cancer Institute. Plans were to establish 20 new endowed chairs in the institute. Other goals of the five-year plan included increased efforts to recruit the nation's finest scientists to the OUHSC campus.

In 2006, Dr. Stephen Prescott became the ninth president of the Oklahoma Medical Research Foundation. Prescott came to OMRF from the University of Utah where he founded its program in human and molecular biology and genetics. In the previous ten years, under the guidance of Dr. J. Donald Capra, OMRF's funding from NIH had increased by more than 200 percent and the number of employees grew from 350 to more than 500. OMRF board chairman Len Cason said, "Our scientists have achieved numerous research milestones in the fields of cardiovascular disease, cancer and immunology, and Alzheimer's and brain diseases."

The OMRF institution Dr. Prescott inherited looked nothing

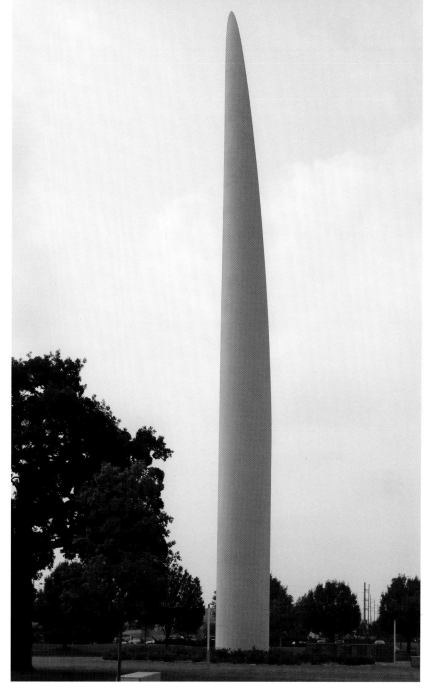

In 2005, the Beacon of Hope, designed by architect Rand Elliott, was dedicated in honor of the 40th anniversary of the founding of the Oklahoma Health Center. The beacon shines each night, emitting a healing light of hope into the sky as a metamorphosis of the human spirit, the will to reach unimaginable heights, and for many whose loved ones are undergoing medical treatment at the OHC institutions. The sculpture, 10 stories high and eight feet wide, pays tribute to the founders of the Oklahoma Health Center, Harvey P. Everest, E.K. Gaylord, Dean A. McGee, Dr. Don O'Donoghue, and Stanton L. Young. *Courtesy Eric Dabney.*

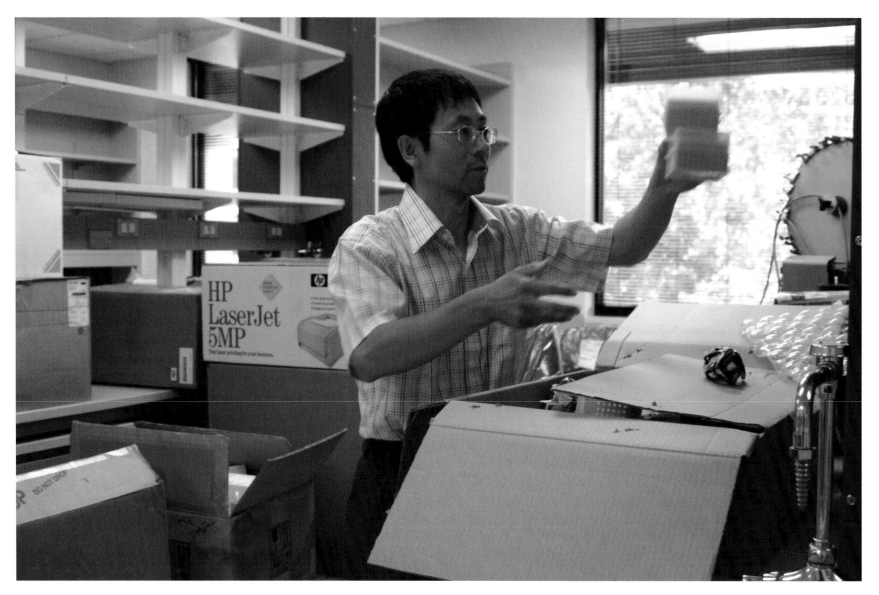

Dr. Zhizhuang Joe Ahao and other researchers moved into laboratory space in the newly completed Phase II of the Stanton L. Young Biomedical Research Center in 2005.
Courtesy OU College of Medicine.

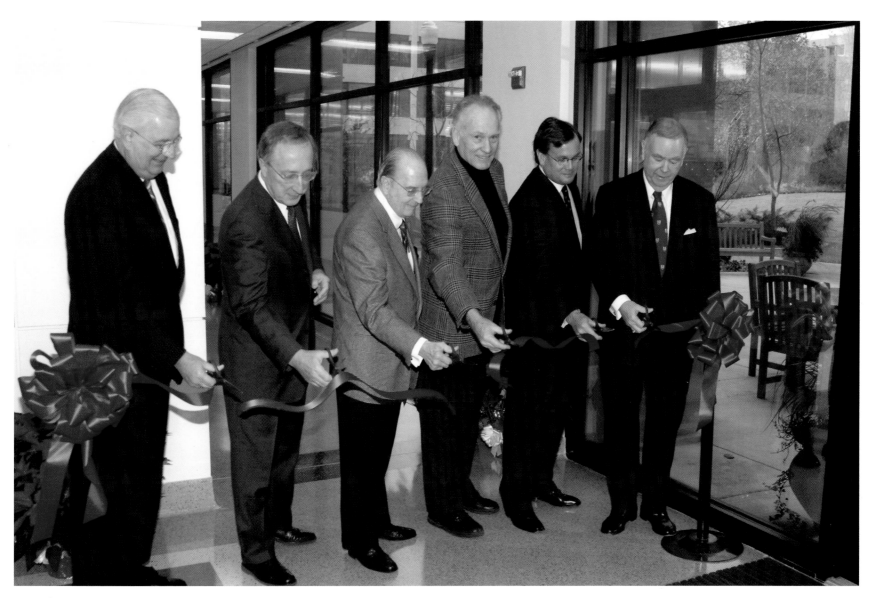

A new $37.9 expansion of the Stanton L. Young Biomedical Research Center opened in December, 2005. At the formal opening are, left to right, OUHSC Provost Dr. Joseph Ferretti, Vice President for Research Dr. Joseph Waner, Stanton L. Young, PHF President Dr. Michael Anderson, University Hospitals Authority and Trust Chairman Michael Samis, and OU President David Boren. *Courtesy OU College of Medicine.*

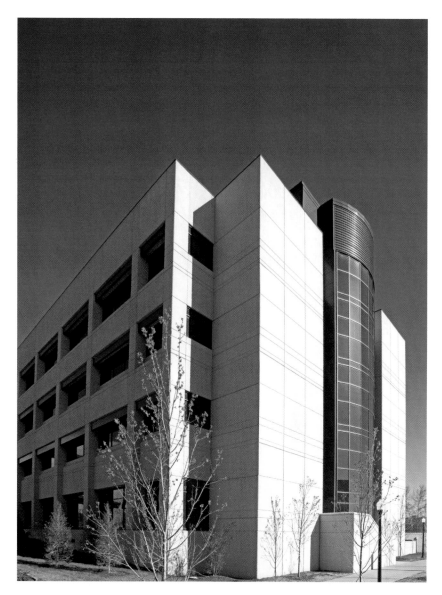

Completion of Phase II of the Stanton L. Young Biomedical Research Center in 2005 increased the size of the center to 233,000 square feet of space dedicated to biomedical, cancer, and genetics research. *Courtesy OU College of Medicine.*

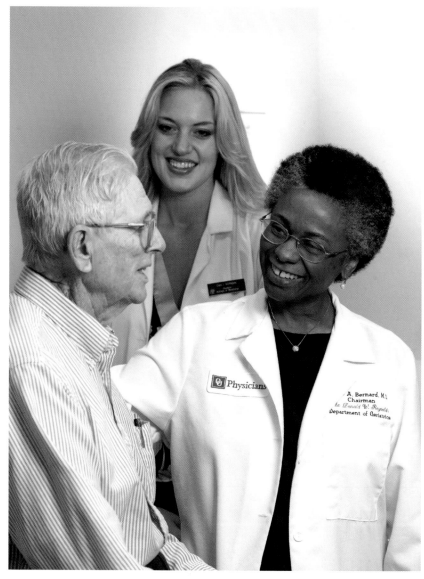

Dr. Marie Bernard, chair of the OU Donald W. Reynolds Department of Geriatric Medicine, visits with a patient as a medical student looks on. Future physicians in the OU College of Medicine are heavily trained in the treatment in care of older Oklahomans. *Courtesy OU College of Medicine.*

like the institution that opened its doors nearly 60 years before. But, in the fast-moving world of medical research, change is the norm. Prescott and his board of directors were confident OMRF was well-positioned to embrace whatever changes and challenges that lay ahead.

In October, 2006, OU President David Boren was a guest editorialist for *The Daily Oklahoman*. Boren predicted the decade "which we are now living" will be the defining decade for Oklahoma. He said, "The actions we take between now and 2010 will shape the quality of life in Oklahoma for the rest of the 21st century."

Boren cited statistics that Oklahoma City was reaping the benefit of a $3 billion impact on the economy from the growth of the biosciences at institutions on the Oklahoma Health Center campus. He called biosciences "the greatest engine for economic diversification." Boren said the state could not afford any delay in recruiting experts to staff the growing research institutions. The OU President called upon the state legislature and private donors to fund the large increase in human talent needed. He said, "Historians will honor them for their actions. Let us vow in this decade we will propel Oklahoma into national leadership for the rest of the century. Oklahomans have the vision and tenacity to do it!"

The Dean McGee Eye Institute (DMEI) broke ground in November, 2006, on a 78,000-square-foot state-of-the-art science laboratory and clinical research and patient care space adjacent to the existing facility built three decades before. More than $30 million had been raised in a capital building campaign for the project doubling the existing space.

Institute President Dr. David Parke II said the expansion would

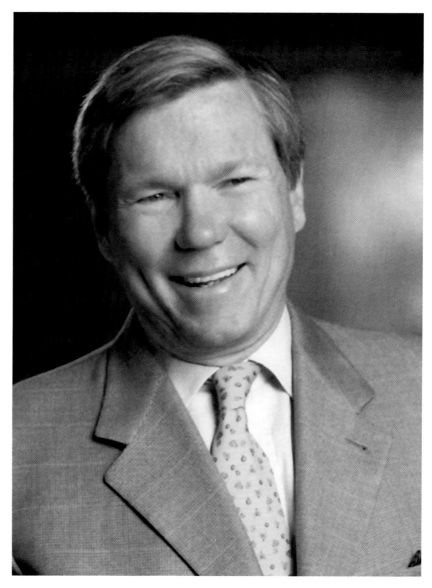

Dr. Stephen Prescott became president of the Oklahoma Medical Research Foundation in 2006. *Courtesy Oklahoma Medical Research Foundation.*

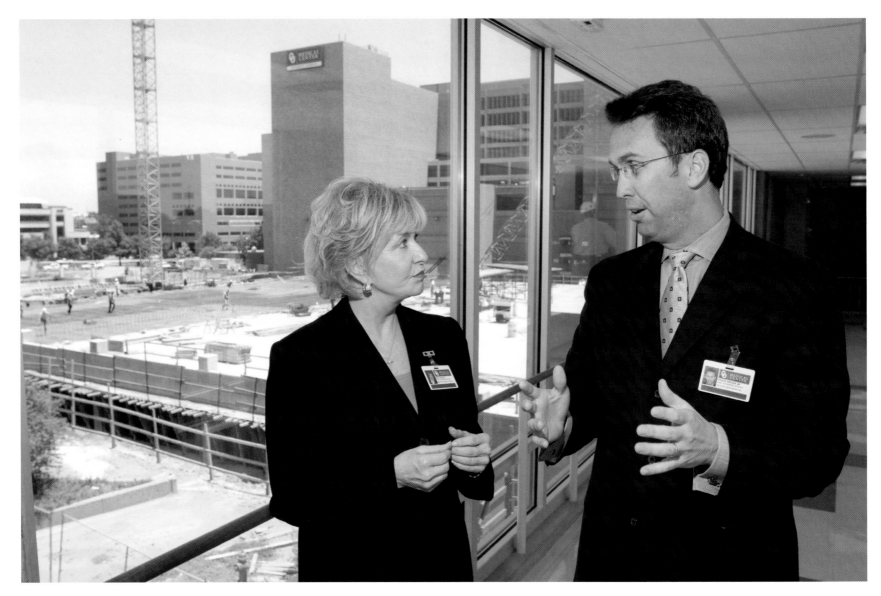

Rebecca Benoit, chief operating officer of Presbyterian Hospital at the OU Medical Center, left, and Chuck Spicer, chief operating officer of Children's Hospital at the OU Medical Center, meet in the walkway between the two towers in 2006. Construction for the new OU Children's Physicians Building can be seen in the background. *Courtesy OU College of Medicine.*

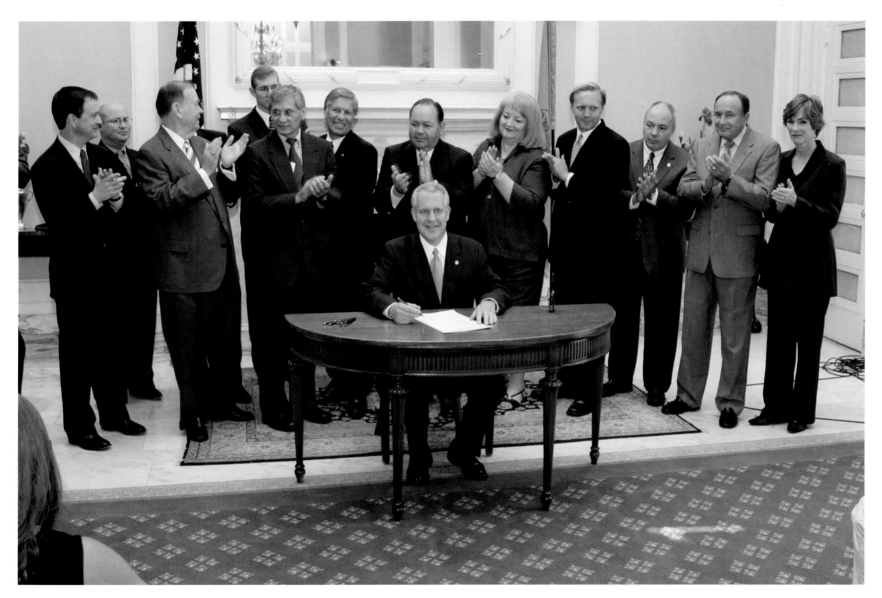

Members of the Oklahoma legislature and other dignitaries applaud after Governor Brad Henry signs legislation to fund development of the Oklahoma Diabetes Center in 2006. Directly behind Governor Henry is Governor Bill Anoatubby of the Chickasaw Nation. To his left is Choctaw Chief Greg Pyle. At the signing, the Chickasaws announced a gift of $2 million to the diabetes center and the Choctaws announced a gift of $1 million. *Courtesy OU College of Medicine.*

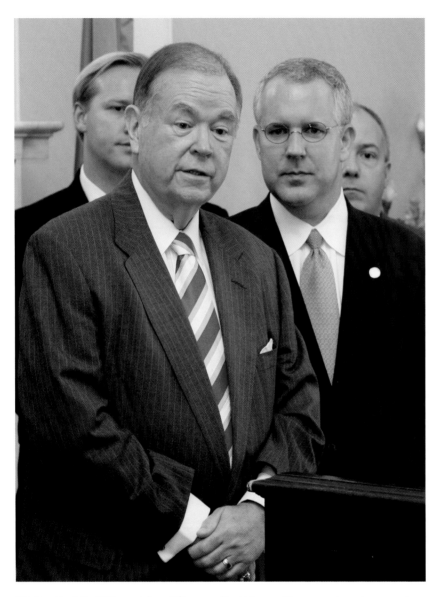

OU President David Boren, left, and Governor Brad Henry address reporters at ceremonies announcing the funding of the Oklahoma Diabetes Center in 2006.
Courtesy OU College of Medicine.

allow the eye institute to add about 100 new employees, including new scientists and physicians. DMEI sees 140,000 patients annually and the expanded facilities will substantially increase the number of patient visits.

DMEI is closely affiliated with the OU College of Medicine. Each medical student spends time at the eye institute, every resident in ophthalmology is based at DMEI, and many DMEI researchers are full-time faculty at the medical school. Parke said, "We have a very tight relationship that we value tremendously, and benefits both parties."

In early 2006, Oklahoma Medical Research Foundation President Dr. J. Donald Capra called upon legislators and state leaders to provide more funding for research. He pointed out Oklahoma, from 2000 to 2004, ranked eighth among the states in the growth of funding from the National Institutes of Health. The bad news was Oklahoma still averaged only $25 per citizen in NIH funding, less than one third the national average.

"The problem is numbers," Dr. Capra said, "OMRF, which represents more than a third of the state's medical research funding, simply doesn't have enough scientists to put our state in the same league with California, which averages about $100 in NIH funding per capita, or even Alabama with $72 per capita average." Dr. Capra said, "Investing in infrastructure today is crucial to stopping heart disease, cancer, and Alzheimer's tomorrow. Indeed, our children's lives may depend on it."

The "no vacancy" sign went up at the PHF Research Park in April, 2006, as the last 1,800 square feet, of nearly 600,000 square feet, was committed. In the previous 20-month period, 24 new tenants had been added, bringing the total to 44. The latest tenant was a company created by OUHSC researcher Dr. Jian-Xing "Jay" Ma

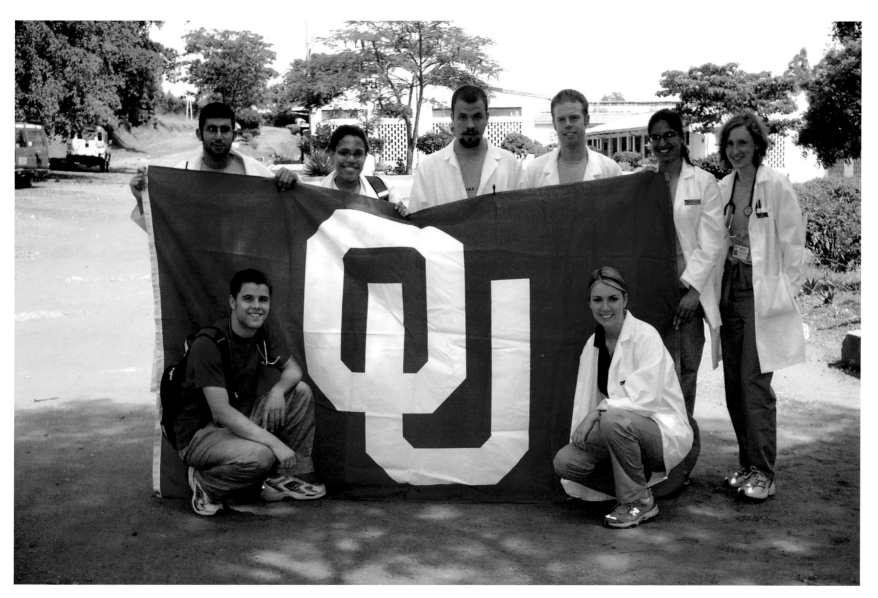

Eight members of the OU College of Medicine's Class of 2009 spent four weeks as volunteers at St. Joseph's Missionary Hospital in Migori Town, Kenya, in the summer of 2006. The trip was made possible by the OU College of Medicine Alumni Association. Left to right, front row, Alexander Williams and Kerri May. Back row, Pedram Behzadi, Christen Flack, Jacob O'Melia, Brett Derrevere, Sunita Chahar, and Heath Mueller. *Courtesy OU College of Medicine.*

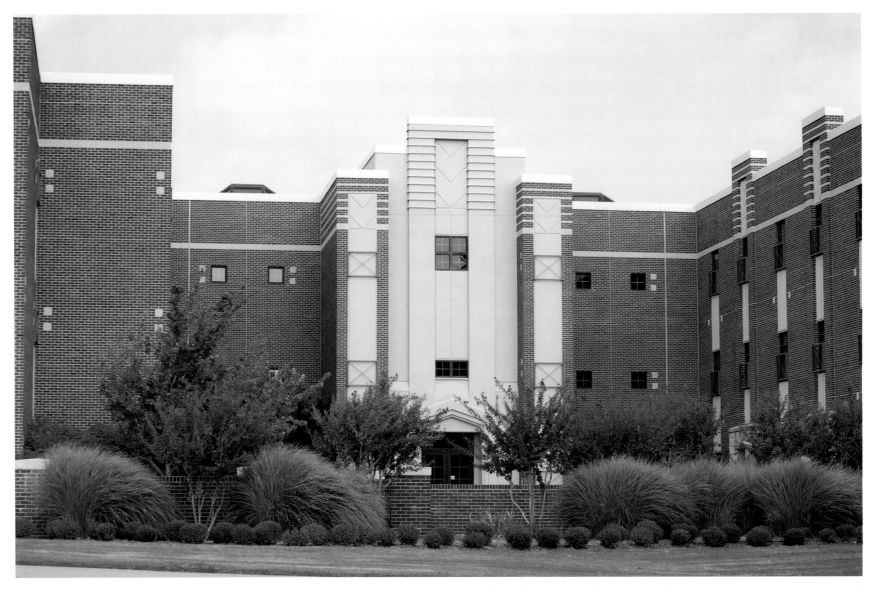

The Oklahoma School of Science and Mathematics campus is a combination of green lawns and beautiful buildings. Inside, Oklahoma's brightest students study under the tutelage of dedicated faculty. The OSSM Classes of 1998 and 2000 achieved the highest ACT composite scores of any high school in the United States. *Courtesy Eric Dabney.*

called Charlesson LLC and its subsidiary, Lifetrees LLC.

By the end of 2006, the Oklahoma Health Center had become one of the nation's largest concentrations of health care services and research. The 300-acre campus had an unbelievable impact upon the economy and was still growing. OU Medical Center's Children's Hospital was involved in a $40 million capital improvement building project, part of $100 million campus-wide construction.

OU President Boren led the effort to create a world-class Oklahoma Diabetes Center. Boren, who was diagnosed with Type 2 diabetes in 2004, predicted that Oklahoma could be in the small handful of top diabetes centers just as the nation slowly wakes up to the diabetes threat and research grants begin flowing. Oklahoma ranks at the top among the states in per capita number of citizens who suffer from diabetes.

In 2006, Boren announced major gifts from the Hille Foundation, Tulsa businessman Henry Zarrow, the Chickasaw and Choctaw nations, and a $9 million appropriation from the state legislature to build an adult facility and a children's diabetes center. The facility will provide comprehensive outpatient diabetes care and education and access to the latest developments in diabetes management and clinical research.

A 2006 study released by the Greater Oklahoma City Chamber of Commerce showed the booming bioscience industry centered on the OHC campus had a direct economic impact of $3.4 billion annually. The study by economists Robert C. Dauffenbach, John McCraw, and Larkin Warner found 44,500 people employed in the state's bioscience industry, with total employment, including spin-off jobs generated by the industry, exceeding 90,000. The study included bioscience employment from hospitals and health care to laboratories and research. The chamber hired the Battelle Institute

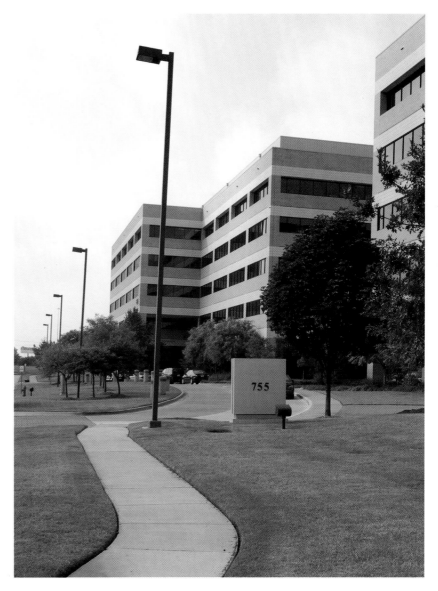

Attractive landscaping tops off major construction at the Presbyterian Health Foundation Research Park. *Courtesy Eric Dabney.*

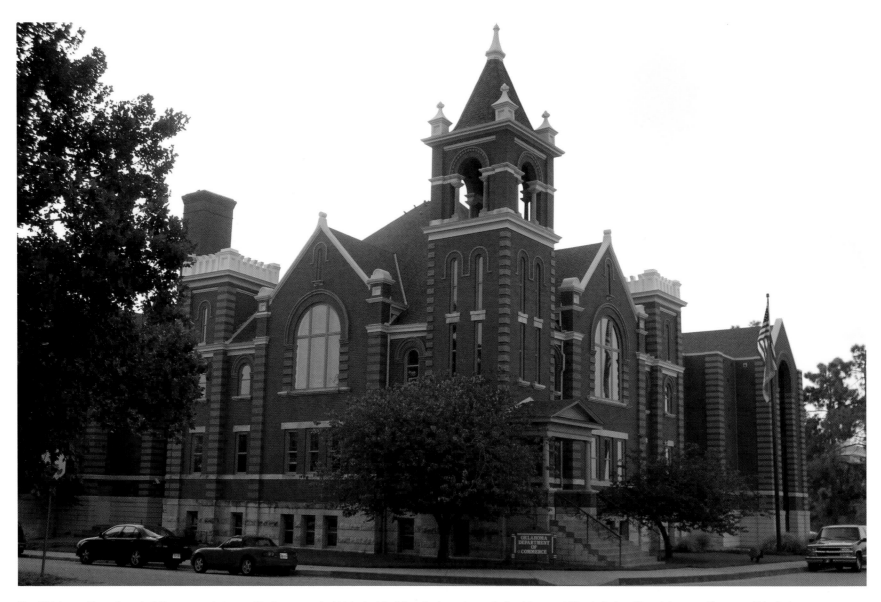

The Oklahoma Department of Commerce is housed in the renovated historical building that was home to the Maywood Presbyterian Church in 1907. *Courtesy Eric Dabney.*

to create a "road map" to build the life sciences industry. The Battelle report identified 14 actions that Oklahoma leaders should take to grow the industry.

OHC Foundation President Hershel Lamirand described the concentration of bioscience efforts on the OHC campus as an example of the "incredible pulling power this complex has." At the time the study was released, PHF President Dr. Michael Anderson announced the construction on a 155,000-square-foot, five-story building, the seventh building in the PHF Research Park.

In 2006, David Wood became the new director of the Oklahoma City Veterans Affairs Medical Center (VAMC) on the OHC campus. It was a time when a national debate was occurring on medical treatment for veterans. Under Wood's direction, the Oklahoma City VAMC implemented several customer service initiatives in 2007. The new programs included patient satisfaction surveys, post-discharge phone calls, patient education programs, and a revamped customer service department. It was part of the national effort to improve the quality of service to the nation's veterans.

As other veterans' hospitals in the nation received criticism, the Oklahoma VAMC was applauded for computerizing its records system to make it easier for the hospital to access patient histories and share information with other doctors and hospitals. The second change giving the Oklahoma City facility high marks was a new approach to set appointments and alleviate long waits that veterans endured in the past.

In April, 2007, Congresswoman Mary Fallin was the keynote speaker for a dedication ceremony of the VAMC's renovated Neurosciences Unit. The 20-bed inpatient unit provides specialized care to veterans with neurological disorders and chronic disabling

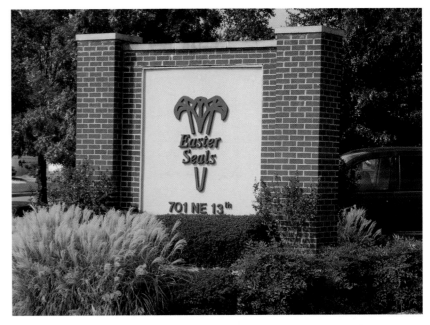

Easter Seals facilities on the OHC campus house a Child Development Center to provide daycare for children with and without special needs, including care for autistic children. An Adult Day Services Program assists families in placing older members in a daycare service. Easter Seals also operates a Medical Rehabilitation Services unit. *Courtesy Eric Dabney.*

disorders. The VAMC in Oklahoma City is greatly aided by volunteers. In 2007, nearly 700 volunteers donated more than 116,000 hours of service.

A unique program at the Oklahoma City VAMC is the chaplain program. Reverend Philip Chapman and four other full-time chaplains conduct baptisms, coordinate religious services, and provide comfort to the thousands of veterans who receive care at the facility each year. The courts have ruled that veterans should have access to their faith tradition even while getting federal health care.

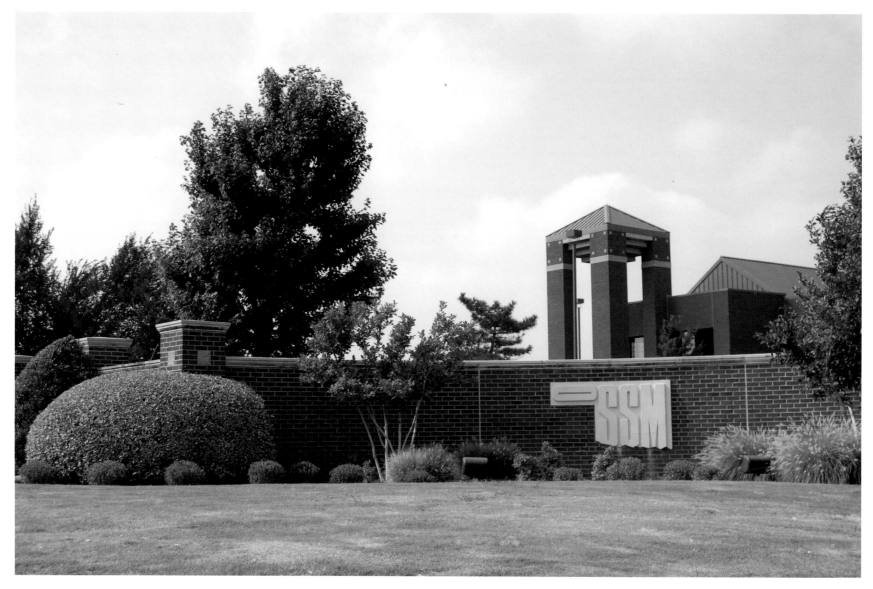

The May 8, 2006 issue of *Newsweek* Magazine named the Oklahoma School of Science and Mathematics one of America's "Elite Public Schools." *Courtesy Eric Dabney.*

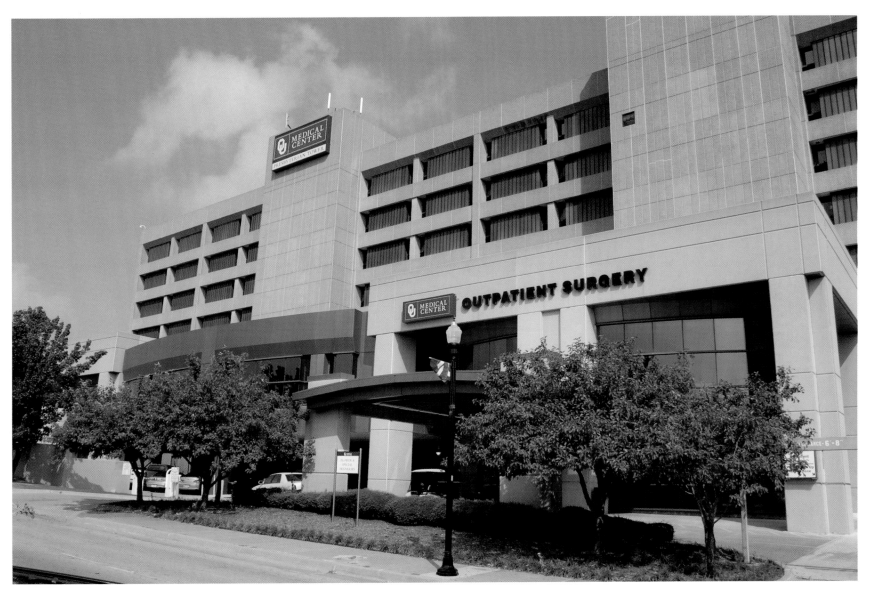

Outpatient surgery has become a major part of services provides by physicians at the OU Medical Center. *Courtesy Eric Dabney.*

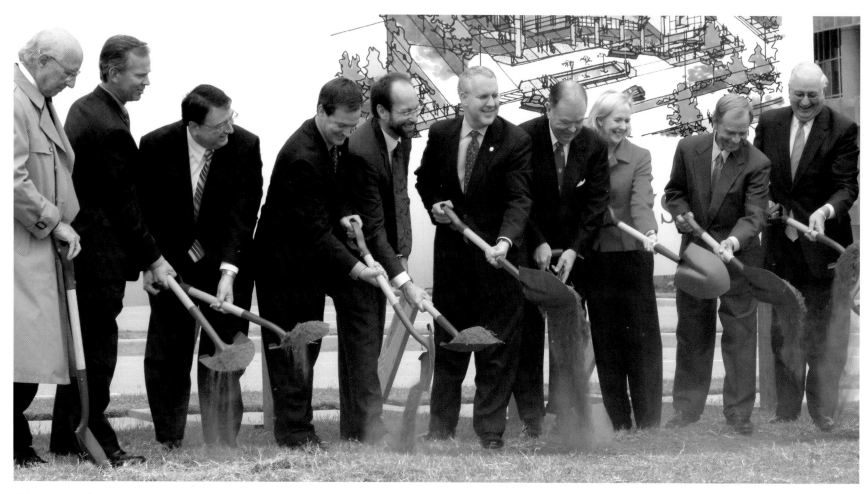

OU and state officials break ground in 2007 for the OU Cancer Institute. Left to right, Banker Gene Rainbolt, OU Regent Dr. John Bell, Medical School Dean Dr. Dewayne Andrews, State Treasurer Scott Meacham, Cancer Institute Director Dr. Robert Mannel, Governor Brad Henry, OU President David Boren, Christy and Jim Everest, co-chairs of the project's fund-raising campaign, and OU Health Sciences Center Provost Dr. Joseph Ferretti. *Courtesy University of Oklahoma.*

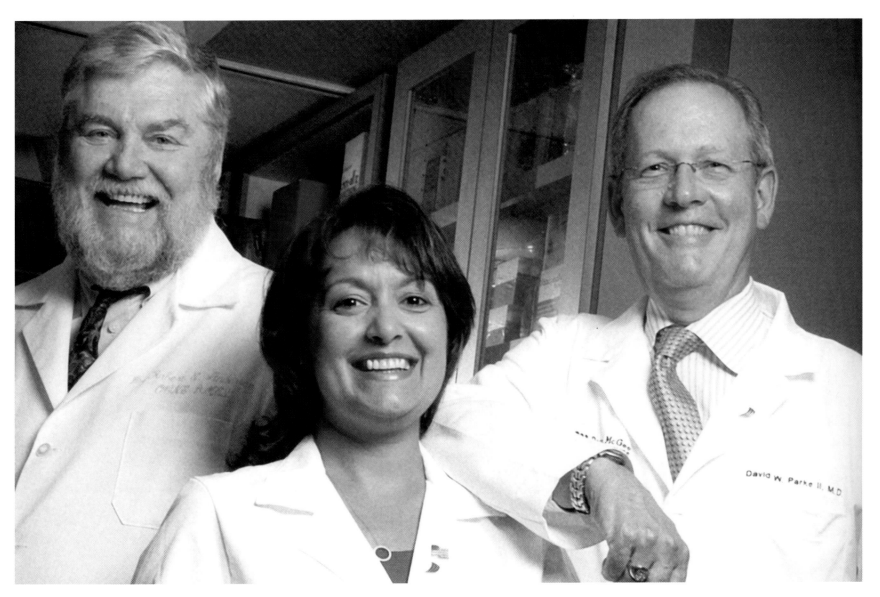

Vision researcher Dr. Michelle Callegan, associate professor of ophthalmology, center, benefits from grants from the National Institutes of Health. At left is Dr. Robert E. "Gene" Anderson, director of research of the Dean McGee Eye Institute and professor of cell biology and ophthalmology at the OU College of Medicine. At right is Dr. David W. Parke II, president and CEO of the eye institute and chair of the OU Department of Ophthalmology. *Courtesy OU College of Medicine.*

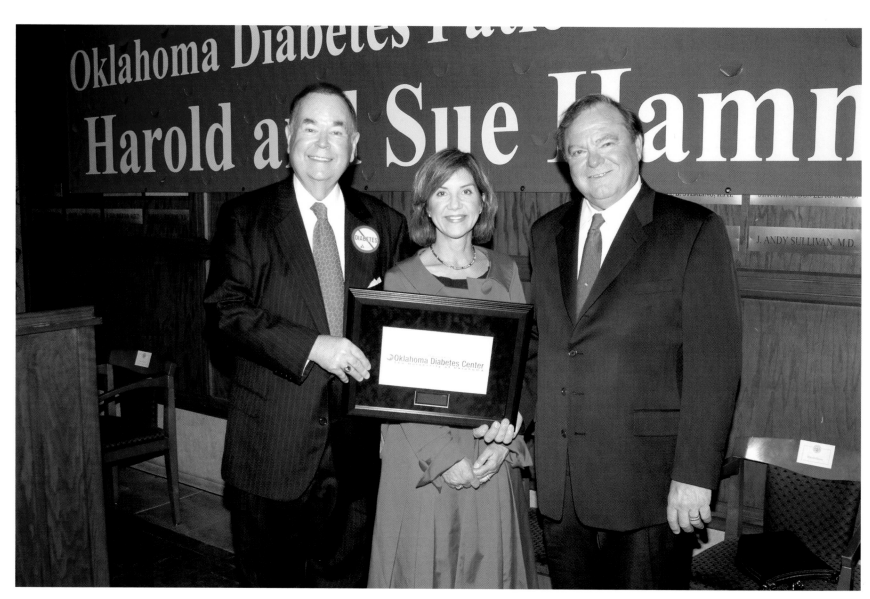

OU President David Boren, left, with Sue and Harold Hamm of Enid. The Hamm Foundation contributed $7 million toward the construction of the Harold Hamm Oklahoma Diabetes Center. *Courtesy University of Oklahoma.*

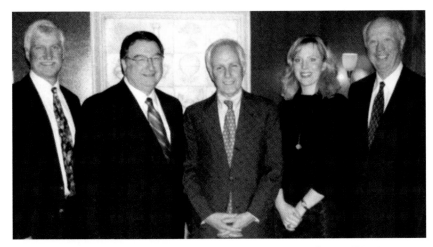

In 2007, Dr. Norman Fost was the first recipient of the Patricia Price Browne Prize in Biomedical Ethics, awarded by the OU College of Medicine and Children's Medical Research Institute. It was named for the late Patricia Browne, a past president and charter member of CMRI. Left to right, Dr. Terrence Stull, chair of the Department of Pediatrics, Dr. M. Dewayne Andrews, dean of the OU College of Medicine, Dr. Fost, and Whitney Browne Hooten and Henry Browne, Patricia Browne's daughter and husband. *Courtesy University of Oklahoma.*

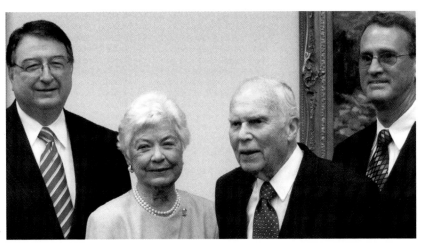

Dr. Donald D. Albers, longtime clinical professor of urology in the OU College of Medicine, was honored in 2007 with the establishment of an endowed chair in his name. Left to right, Dean M. Dewayne Andrews, Mignon Albers, Dr. Albers, and Dr. Daniel Culkin, chairman of the Department of Urology. *Courtesy University of Oklahoma.*

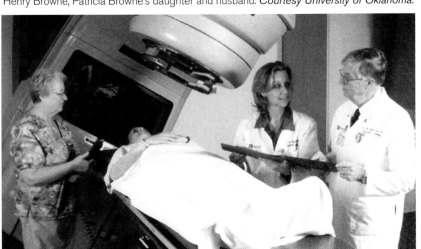

Left to right, chief therapist Joanna Ingram, Dr. Elizabeth J. Syzek, and Dr. Carl Bogardus are part of the new emphasis on treatment of cancer at the Oklahoma Medical Center. *Courtesy OU Medical Center.*

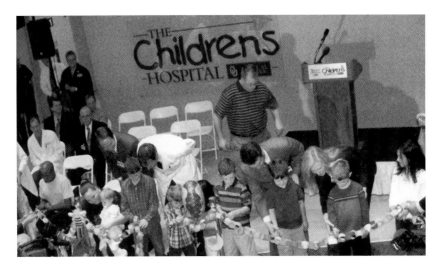

Young patients prepare to cut a paper chain to officially open Everett Tower as the new Children's Hospital at OU Medical Center in January, 2007. The opening concluded a $100 million construction project to consolidate pediatric and women's services in the new Children's Hospital, and adult services and the Level 1Trauma Center at Presbyterian Tower. *Courtesy University of Oklahoma.*

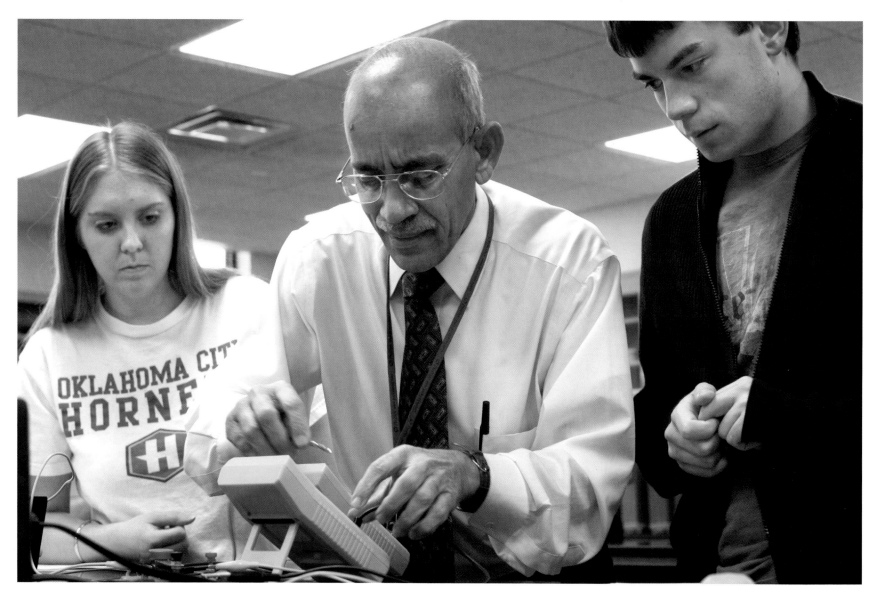

Teacher Jay Rudra demonstrates Ohm's Law to students Amanda Cook, left, and Alex Perry at the Oklahoma School of Science and Mathematics. *Courtesy Oklahoma Publishing Company.*

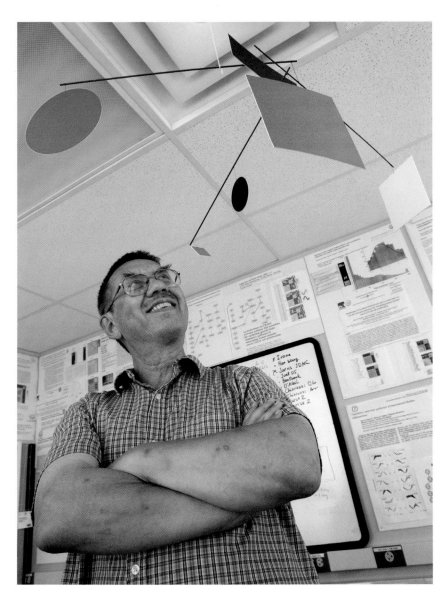

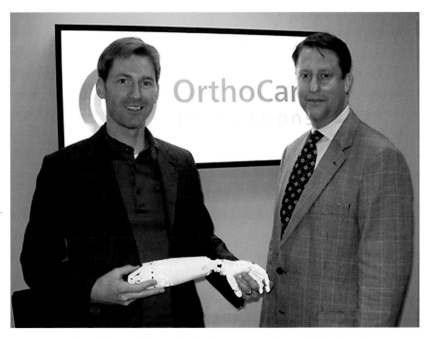

Jay Martin, left, and Doug McCormack, chief executive officer of OrthoCare Innovations, show off a prototype of a prosthetic hand in the company's Oklahoma headquarters in the Presbyterian Health Foundation Research Park. *Courtesy Oklahoma Publishing Company.*

Igor Dozmorov, director of bioinformatics at the microarray research facility of the Oklahoma Medical Research Foundation, looks at a mobile hanging in his office that he uses to represent human genes and the relationships between each of them. *Courtesy Oklahoma Publishing Company.*

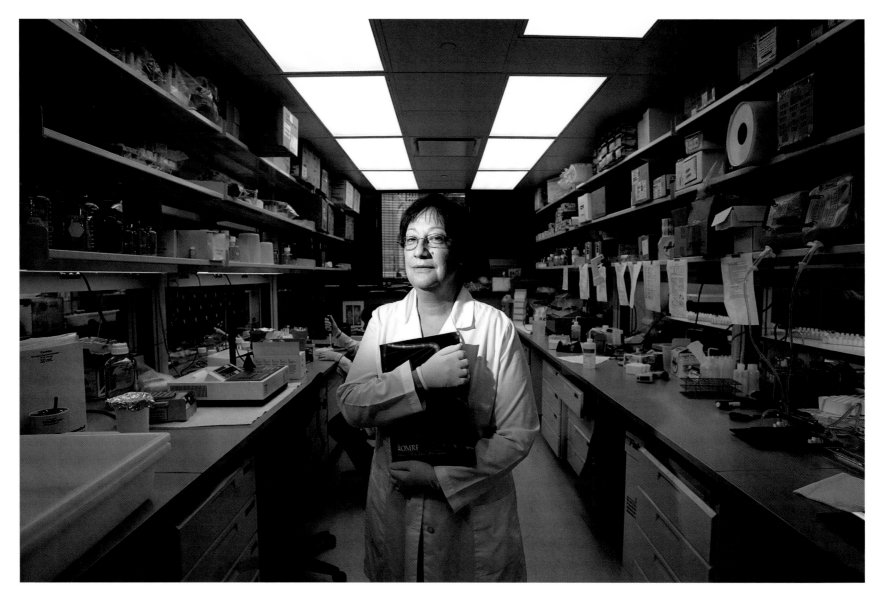

Joan Merrill, head of Clinical Pharmacology R   esearch at the Oklahoma Medical Research Foundation, is shown in her laboratory in 2006. *Courtesy Oklahoma Publishing Company.*

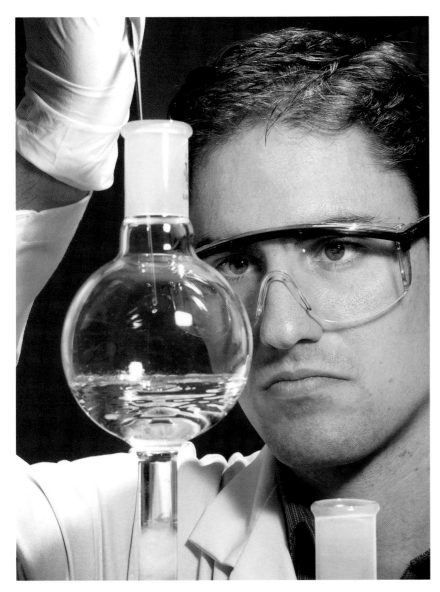

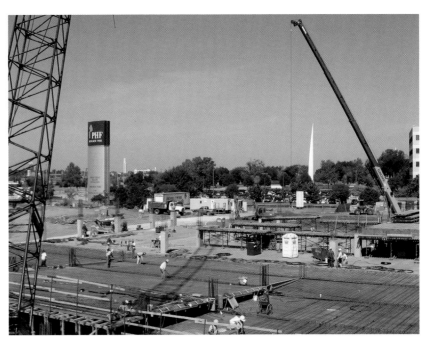

Construction cranes frame the progress of construction at the PHF Research Park in 2006. *Courtesy Oklahoma Publishing Company.*

Geoff Bilcer, director of Medicinal Chemistry at Zapaq, Inc., demonstrates a routine lab function in purifying productions in the company's laboratory at the PHF Research Park. *Courtesy Oklahoma Publishing Company.*

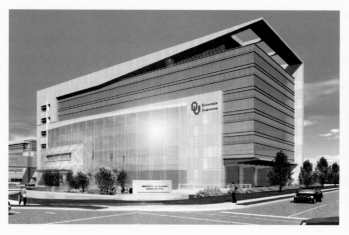
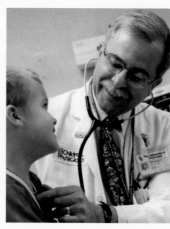
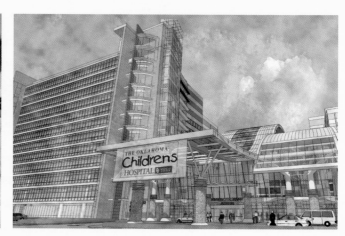

Chapter Ten

A Bright Future

A master plan released by the Oklahoma Health Center in 2007 predicted that expansion on the campus could mean as much as $1.48 billion in construction by 2022. Thousands of hours were spent developing the plan for campus expansion to help meet the health needs of Oklahomans. It is anticipated 4.75 million square feet will be added by 2022.

The OHC Master Plan was the vision of Dr. M. Dewayne Andrews, dean of the OU College of Medicine, and the leaders and staffs of OHC institutions. Coordination of the project came from Miles Associates/HOK Planning Group and Tom Godkins, OUHSC Associate Vice President for Facilities Management and Director of Capital Planning.

OHCF President Hershel Lamirand said some property acquisition would be necessary if the expansion goes as planned, but residential properties will not be affected. The plan calls for empty areas to be filled and older buildings razed to make way for higher density structures.

The principal objectives of the OHC Master Plan are:

- Establish the OHC as the primary destination for health care and education;
- Achieve a campus that supports the missions and strategic goals of the OHC;
- Increase the OHC's status as a major economic engine for the region.

At the time the 2007 Master Plan was unveiled, four major projects were under construction at a cost of more than $84 million and 13 other projects worth $180 million had been funded, but were not yet under construction. Planners projected 38 projects within five years at a cost of $616 million, 26 projects from five to ten years out, costing $403 million, and 11 long-term projects that would cost nearly $200 million.

The planned projects cover a broad range of health care, education, research, housing, and infrastructure. Terry Taylor, OHCF Director of Planning and Operations, said, "The most intensive growth is focused toward patient care, academics, and research in the core of the existing campus, and is driven primarily

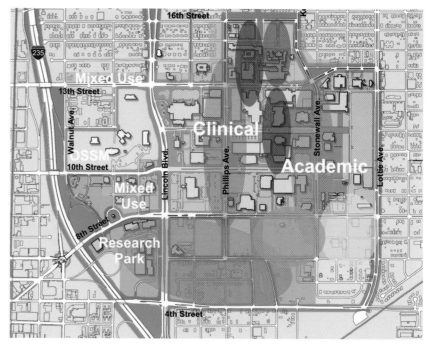

The Oklahoma Health Center Master Plan in 2007 identifies distinct subdivision within the OHC campus. *Courtesy Oklahoma Health Center Foundation.*

by the vigorous expansion of the College of Medicine."

Twenty nine future projects are planned in the area known as the Clinical Corridor, Phillips Avenue between Northeast 6th and 13th streets. The plan also projects the parking needs of OHC to grow by 14,000 spaces, an 83 percent increase over current capacity. The plan encourages the use of public transportation to reduce parking spaces that must be built in multi-level facilities.

The master plan extends the popular broad and meaningful green spaces on the campus with gardens, water features, paths, and benches woven among buildings. Eventually, planners want

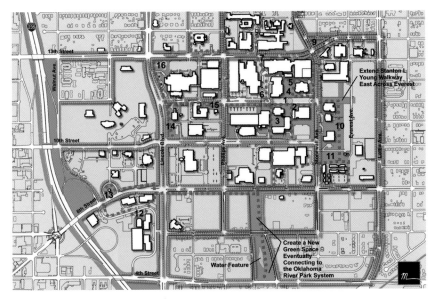

Walking paths are a desired concept in the Oklahoma Health Center Master Plan adopted in 2007 to carry the Oklahoma Health Center campus forward to 2022. *Courtesy Oklahoma Health Center Foundation.*

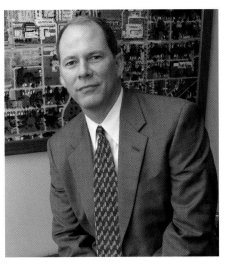

Director of Planning and Operations Terry Taylor's primary responsibilities include guiding the growth of the OHC, solidifying its boundaries and promoting planned development. *Courtesy Mark Harmon and OKCBusiness Magazine.*

the campus to link the Oklahoma River by pedestrian, bicycle, and vehicle routes. There are also plans for connected pathways to new housing projects along I-235, Bricktown, downtown Oklahoma City, and the State Capitol area. Taylor said, "Within this framework, growth and development can occur with purpose and order."

Even as planners put their dreams on paper, progress continued on several fronts within the OHC family of institutions. In 2007, Easter Seals Oklahoma, Inc., operated child development and adult day services programs from its headquarters on the OHC campus. The organization was formerly known as the Oklahoma Society for Crippled Children. On any given week, Easter Seals Oklahoma has 75 children and 40 adults enrolled in the programs.

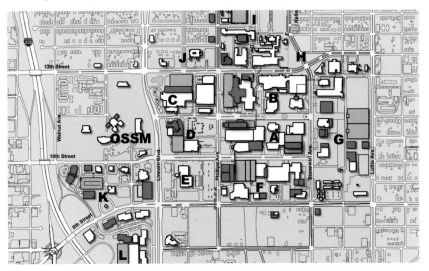

Planned development on the Oklahoma Health Center campus through 2022 are indicated in red. Every few years, OHC principals gather to plan for orderly development of the area. *Courtesy Oklahoma Health Center Foundation.*

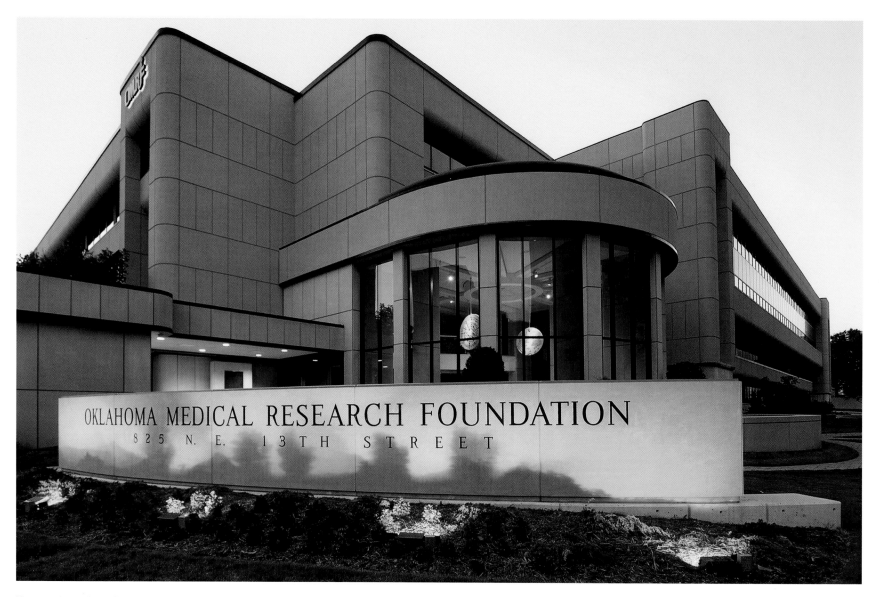

The new look of the Oklahoma Medical Research Foundation headquarters after new construction began in 2008. *Courtesy Oklahoma Medical Research Foundation.*

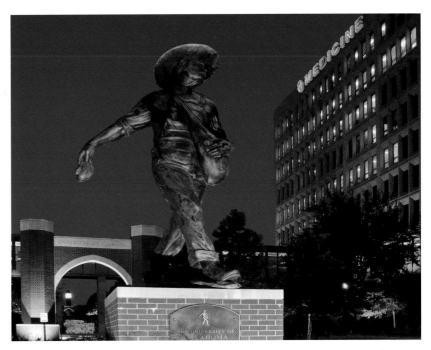

Paul Moore's "The Seed Sower" is an important part of OUHSC beautification efforts of OU First Lady Molly Boren. In the background is the Biomedical Sciences Building. *Courtesy OU College of Medicine.*

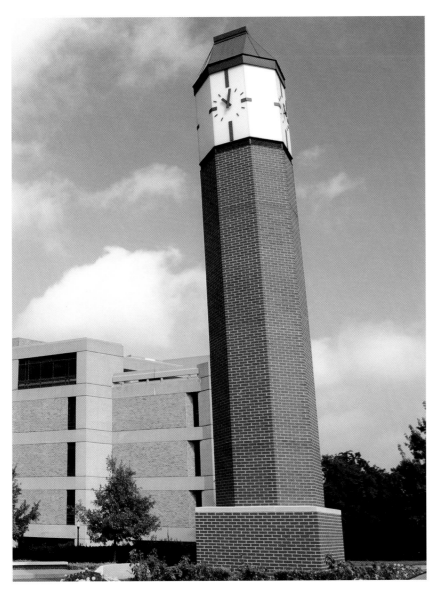

Part of the OUHSC beautification project, the Thelma Gaylord Memorial Clock Tower is seen through the Mothers' Garden. *Courtesy OU College of Medicine.*

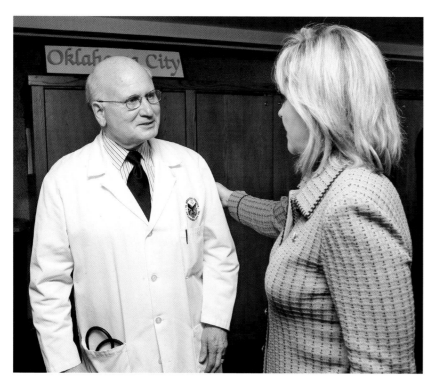

Congresswoman Mary Fallin, right, visits with Dr. Robert McCaffree at the VA Medical Center in 2007. Fallin has been extremely supportive of efforts to bring more federal dollars to the OHC campus. *Courtesy Oklahoma Publishing Company.*

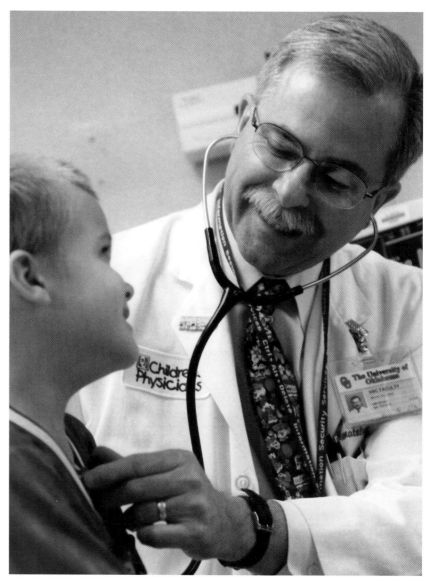

A young cancer patient is examined by Dr. William H. Meyer, director of the Jimmy Everest Center for Cancer and Blood Disorders. Dr. Meyer holds the Children's Medical Research Institute–Ben Johnson Chair in Hematology-Oncology. *Courtesy OU College of Medicine.*

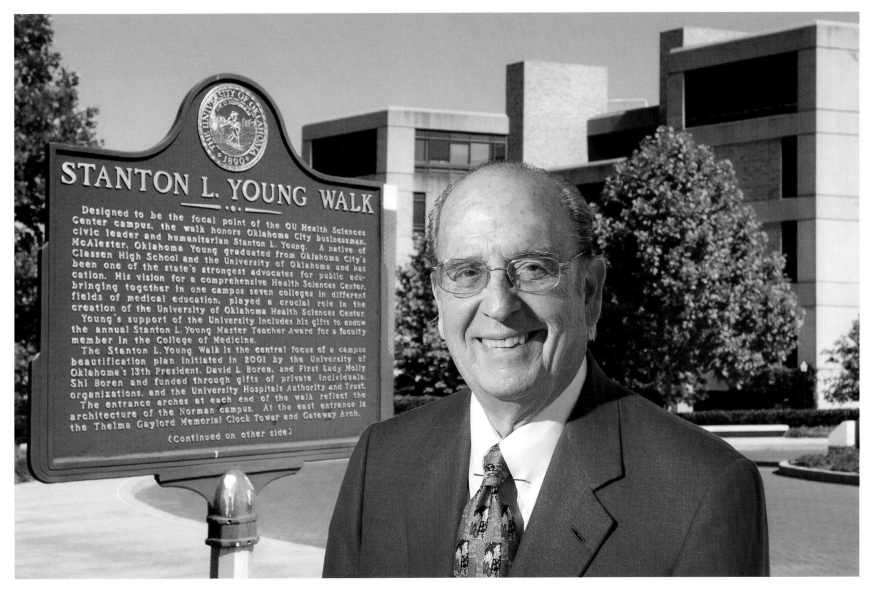

Stanton L. Young has watched the Oklahoma Health Center grow from an idea among Oklahoma City civic leaders to a world-class medical treatment and research center.
Courtesy Oklahoma Publishing Company.

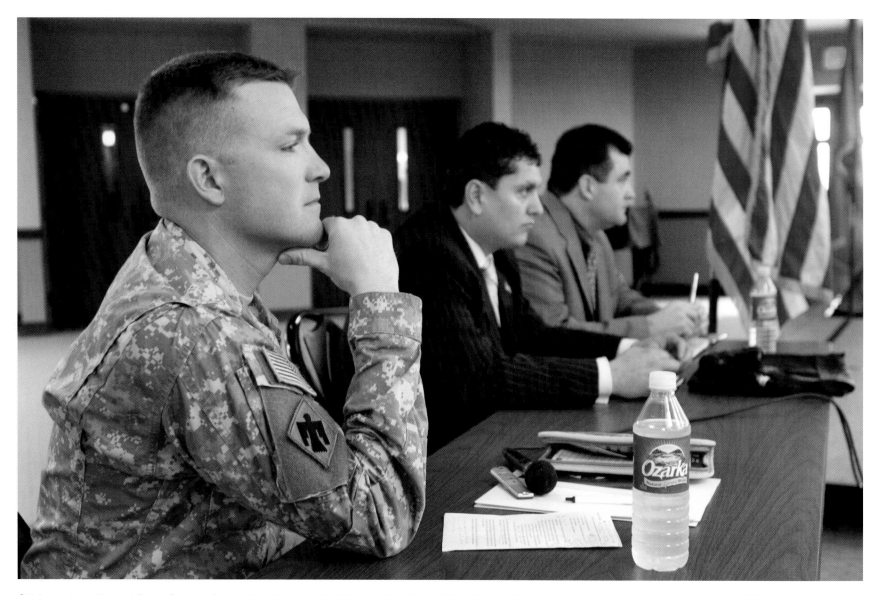

Oklahoma Army National Guard Chaplain Captain Brad Hanna, left, Ed Pulido of the United Way of Central Oklahoma, and Steve Buck, executive director of NAMI Oklahoma, Inc., participate in an emergency summit in 2007 on the mental health needs of Oklahoma's veterans. The summit was co-sponsored by the Oklahoma Department of Mental Health and Substance Abuse Services. *Courtesy Oklahoma Publishing Company.*

In May, 2007, researchers Michael Dresser, Michael Conrad, Emma Lee, and Joseph Wilkerson discovered a gene that controls where chromosomes in the human body go during cell division, a process that could lead to more understanding about Down syndrome and other genetic disorders. The announcement was made by Phillip Silverman, a cell biologist for OMRF's Molecular, Cell, and Developmental Biology Research Program. Silverman said, "I do not claim this discovery will cure a disease, but I can say with complete confidence this will give us new insight into some of these genetic problems."

In September, 2007, Governor Brad Henry presented a $15 million check from the Oklahoma Opportunity Fund to OMRF to serve as seed money for an ambitious $125 million expansion plan that includes an eight-story research tower and 300 new jobs on the OHC campus. The Oklahoma Opportunity Fund was created by the state legislature the year before to help bring new jobs and businesses to the state by providing seed capital. Construction on a new 195,000-square-foot tower north of the present OMRF research facility began in 2008.

In 2008, the Oklahoma BioScience Association (OKBio) was created to carry the vision of bioscience in Oklahoma and become a unified voice for the state's bioscience industry. PHF Board Chairman Carl Edwards was named chairman of the new group's board of directors. Sheri Stickley, deputy director of the Oklahoma Department of Commerce, served as executive liaison for the new organization. She said, "The purpose of OKBio is to build the image of Oklahoma as a bioscience leader and build productive partnerships, a strong research base, and commercialization."

An avid supporter of the formation of OKBio was Craig Shimasaki, president of InterGenetics. He said, "OKBio is the

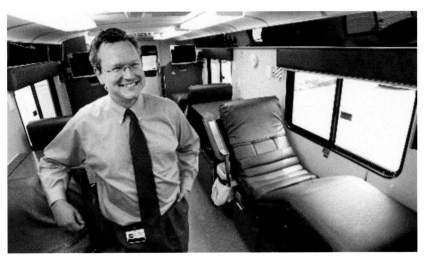

Dr. John Armitage, president of the Oklahoma Blood Institute, in a mobile blood donation unit used to make it easier for Oklahomans to give life-saving plasma. *Courtesy Oklahoma Blood Institute.*

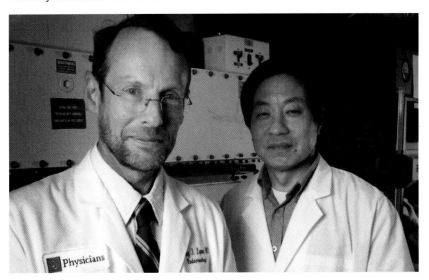

Dr. Timothy J. Lyons, left, holds the Warren Chair in Diabetes Research and directs the Harold Hamm Oklahoma Diabetes Center that received an $11 million grant from the National Institutes of Health in 2007. Jian-xing "Jay" Ma, M.D., Ph.D., right, holds the Laureate Chair in Molecular Medicine and is principal investigator for the grant. *Courtesy OU College of Medicine.*

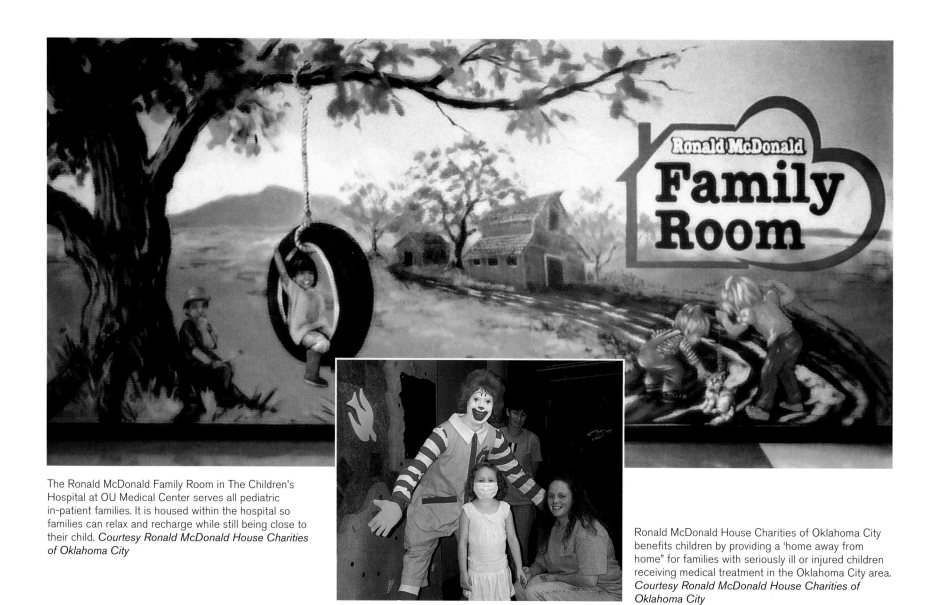

The Ronald McDonald Family Room in The Children's Hospital at OU Medical Center serves all pediatric in-patient families. It is housed within the hospital so families can relax and recharge while still being close to their child. *Courtesy Ronald McDonald House Charities of Oklahoma City*

Ronald McDonald House Charities of Oklahoma City benefits children by providing a 'home away from home" for families with seriously ill or injured children receiving medical treatment in the Oklahoma City area. *Courtesy Ronald McDonald House Charities of Oklahoma City*

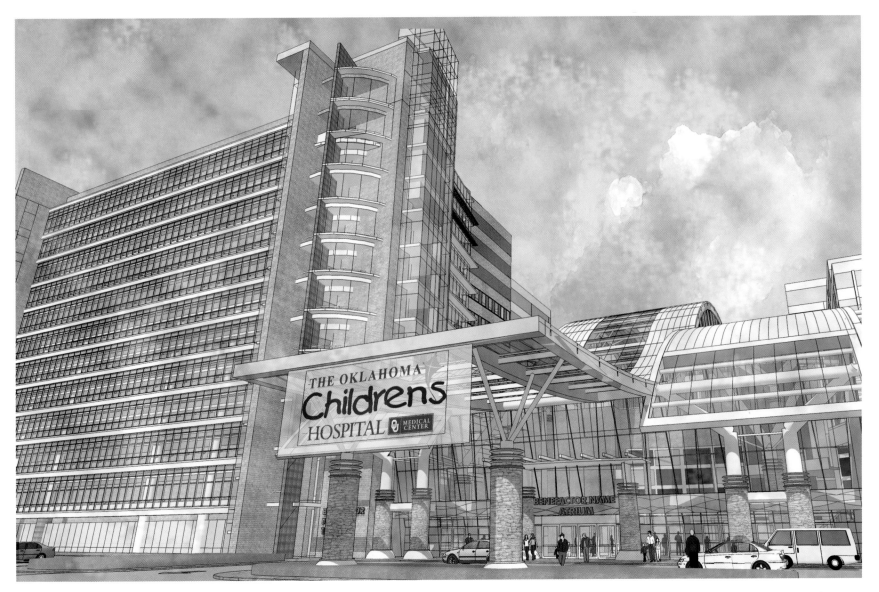

The proposed OU Children's Physicians Building will house the largest pediatric multi-specialty clinic in Oklahoma. A six-story glass and steel atrium will serve as a spectacular entrance to the new building and Children's Hospital at the OU Medical Center. The construction is part of a $110 million project by the University Hospitals Authority and Trust that includes a parking garage and an education center with conference rooms and a 250-seat auditorium. *Courtesy University Hospitals Authority and Trust.*

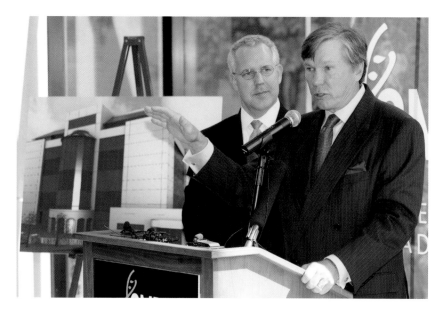

Oklahoma Medical Research Foundation President Dr. Stephen Prescott, right, accepts a $15 million from Governor Brad Henry in 2007 for a $125 million research expansion. *Courtesy Oklahoma Publishing Company.*

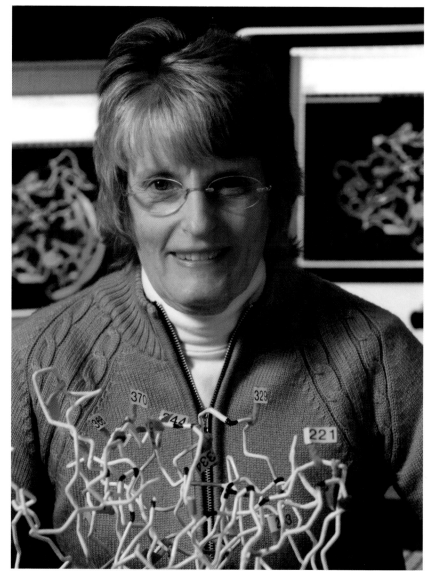

Dr. Gillian Air poses with a 1980s model of an influenza enzyme. Dr. Air and colleagues were first to determine the shape of the enzyme which led to the development of two antiviral drugs. A modern ribbon diagram of the enzyme appears on the monitors behind Dr. Air. *Courtesy OU College of Medicine.*

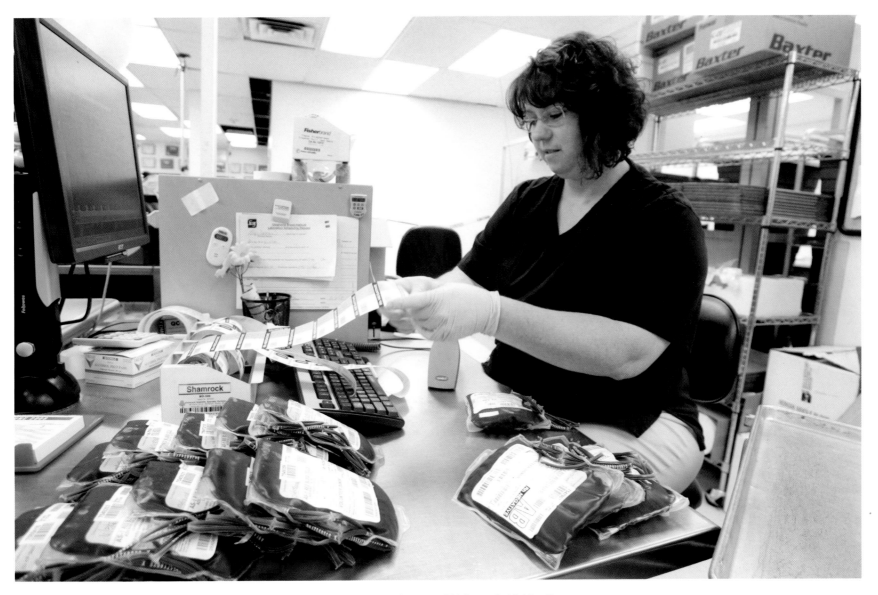

Laboratory technician Carrie Curtis labels blood at the Oklahoma Blood Institute. *Courtesy Oklahoma Publishing Company.*

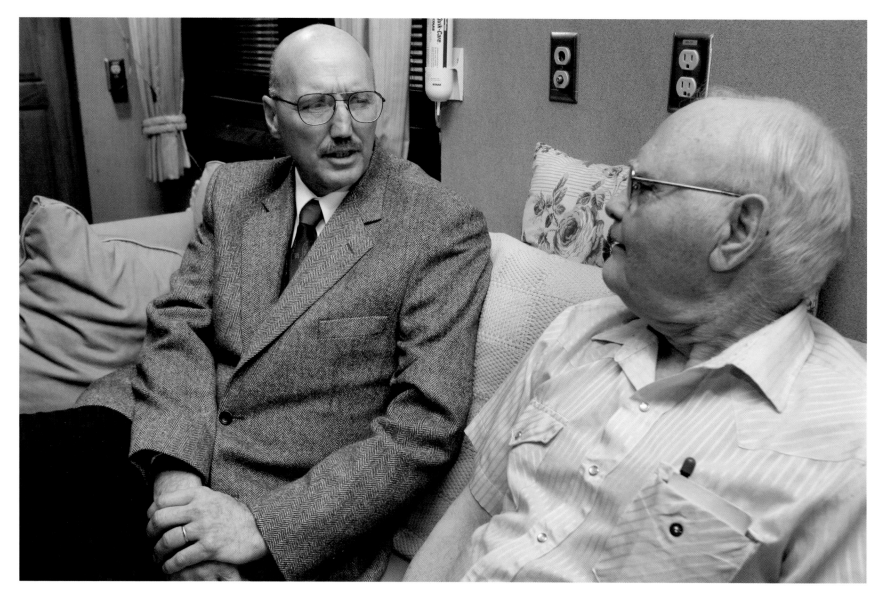

Chaplain Philip Chapman, left, talks with patient Floyd Warren at the Veterans Affairs Medical Center on the OHC campus. *Courtesy Oklahoma Publishing Company.*

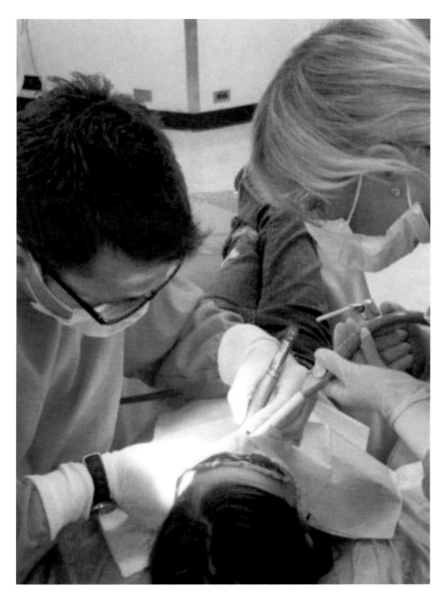

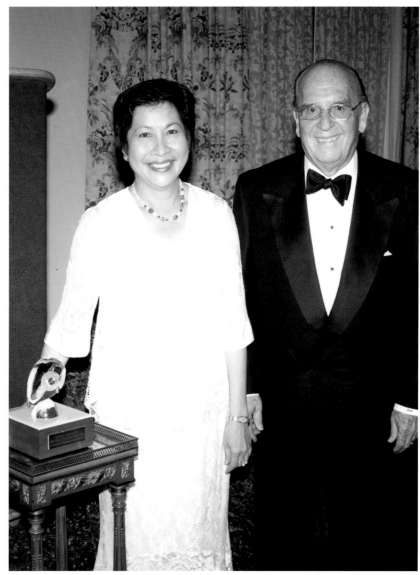

Zane Weaver, left, and Blaire Bowers, OU College of Dentistry students, provide free dental care at the College's 11th annual Kids' Day clinic in 2008. *Courtesy University of Oklahoma.*

Siribhinya Benyahati, left, was honored by Stanton L. Young as the 2007 Stanton L. Young Master Teacher. Established in 1983 through an endowment made by Young, the $15,000 award, one of the largest in the nation for medical teaching excellence, is given annually to a faculty member in the College of Medicine. *Courtesy Oklahoma Health Center Foundation.*

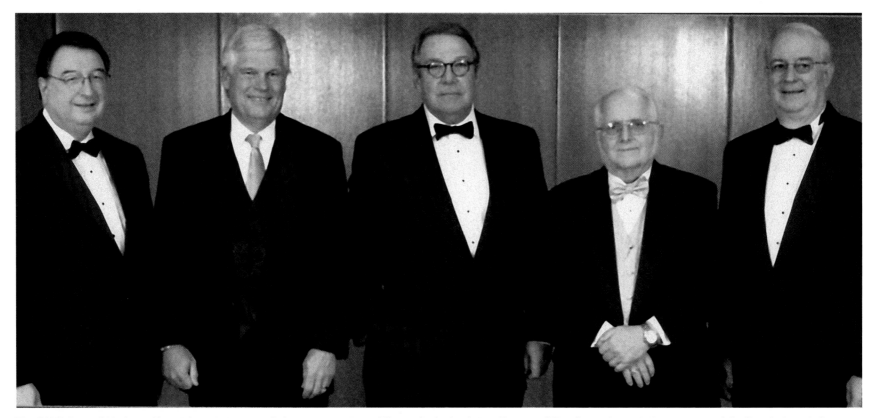

The OU College of Medicine Alumni Association annually honors supporters of the medical school at an Evening of Excellence. In 2008, the recipients of the Dean's Awards for Distinguished Service were presented to Oklahoma City civic leader Carl Edwards, former chair of the Department of Psychiatry and Behavioral Sciences Dr. Gordon Deckert, and the Samuel Roberts Noble Foundation. Left to right, medical school Dean Dr. M. Dewayne Andrews, Edwards, Noble Foundation President Michael Cawley, Dr. Deckert, and OU Health Sciences Center Provost Joseph J. Ferretti. *Courtesy OU College of Medicine.*

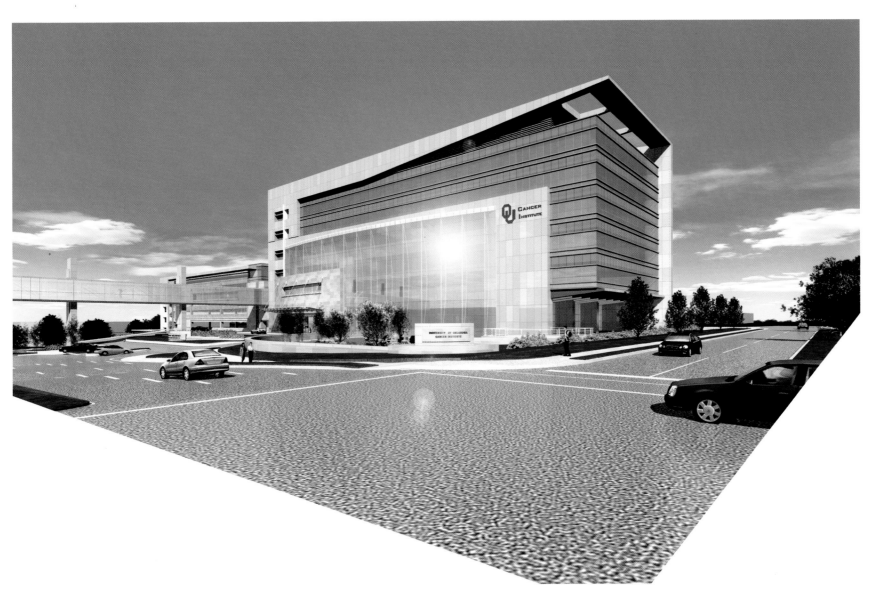

The architect's drawing of the $120 million OU Cancer Institute building scheduled for opening in 2009. A project spearheaded by Provost Ferretti in 1998, OU President David Boren hopes no Oklahoman will ever have to leave the state to receive the latest cancer treatment. *Courtesy OU College of Medicine.*

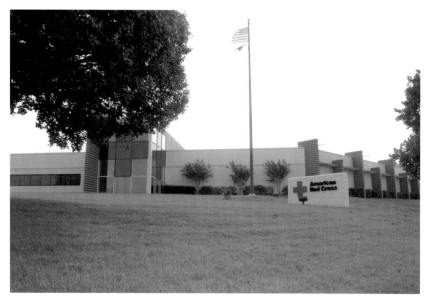

The American Red Cross of Central Oklahoma's headquarters is on the Oklahoma Health Center campus at Northeast Sixth Street and Lincoln Boulevard. When disaster strikes, Red Cross staff and volunteers provide emergency relief to those affected. The Red Cross also provides health and safety education courses. *Courtesy Eric Dabney.*

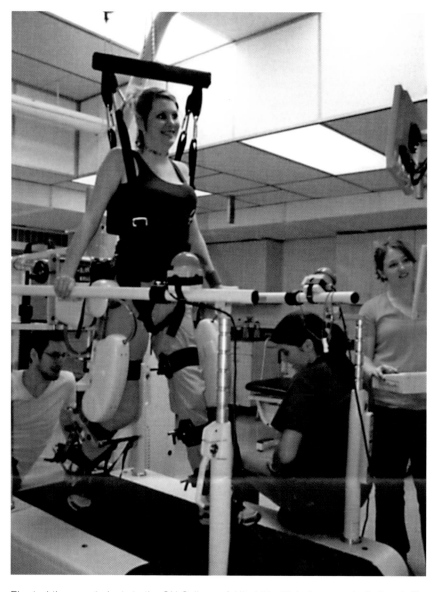

Physical therapy students in the OU College of Allied Health train on a robotic treadmill. OU is one of the few schools in the nation to offer training and therapy on robotic equipment. *Courtesy OUHSC.*

culmination of several steps steadily moving the bioscience industry since our legislature took the bold step in 1987 to pass the Economic Development Act." Shimasaki, quoting Oklahoma's favorite son, Will Rogers, about the constant change of weather in the state, told a reporter, "Oklahoma is a state of change. So it won't be surprising to see another transformation—the emergence of a nationally recognized Oklahoma biotechnology industry producing life-saving drugs, tests, and medical services impacting millions around the world, so that more may live longer, healthier lives."

An example of the magnetism created by the exciting work being accomplished on the OHC campus was Scott Rollins' return to the Sooner State in 2008. Rollins built a $3 billion company based on technology he developed at the Oklahoma Medical Research Foundation and returned to Oklahoma to become president of Selexys Pharmaceuticals, a company attempting to commercialize treatments for inflammatory disease based on research developed by Dr. Rodger McEver at OMRF and Dr. Richard Cummings at OUHSC. Rollins was encouraged to return to his roots by Project Boomerang, an Oklahoma Department of Commerce initiative that targets Oklahoma natives and people with strong ties to the state to bring their skills home.

In the summer of 2008, the Greater Oklahoma City Chamber of Commerce released an economic impact study confirming the PHF Research Park's resounding positive impact upon Oklahoma's economy. Larkin Warner, OSU professor emeritus, and Robert Dauffenbach, associate dean of the Price College of Business at OU, co-authored the study validating the research park had an annual direct economic impact on the economy of $93.6 million, with 1,300 people employed in more than 30 bioscience companies and 20 related entities located in the 27-acre park.

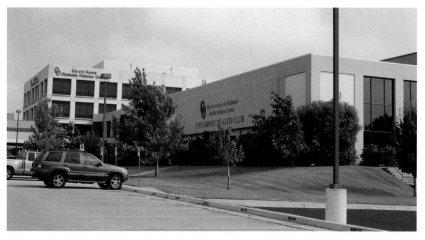

The Harold Hamm Oklahoma Diabetes Center and the University Health Club occupy space originally built by Presbyterian Hospital as a Center for Healthy Living. *Courtesy Eric Dabney.*

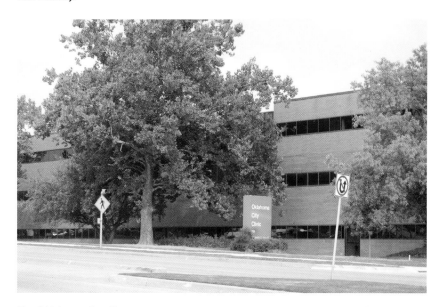

The Oklahoma City Clinic continues as a integral private practice provider of health care on the Oklahoma Health Center campus. The physician group was founded in 1919. *Courtesy Eric Dabney.*

Warner and Dauffenbach wrote, "The park has provided a site for local scientists to take advantage of recent science-driven changes in the structure of the pharmaceutical industry permitting the entry of small biotech enterprises. The park also serves, de facto, as an Oklahoma City accelerator for these firms and provides incubator space."

Oklahoma City Chamber of Commerce President Roy Williams said the study highlighted the benefits of an asset some people may take for granted. "The thing people may quickly overlook," Williams said, "is the fact of how unique it is to have a facility like that in your city, and how it separates us from so many communities. It's a rarity and quite a jewel for Oklahoma."

Proof that local research was being rewarded in commercialization came in 2008 when a Japanese pharmaceutical firm invested $760 million in OMRF's Dr. Jordan Tang's creation of treatment for Alzheimer's disease. OMRF owns the original patents of the products that hopefully can be approved and marketed to millions of Americans afflicted with Alzheimer's.

There are many more commercial success stories in the PHF Research Park. The Oklahoma work of Genzyme, one of the world's leading biotechnology companies, is led by Dr. William Canfield. The company's products are focused on rare inherited disorders, kidney disease, orthopedics, cancer, transplant, immune diseases, and diagnostic testing. Canfield founded Novazyme Pharmaceuticals which was purchased by Genzyme for $200 million. Canfield is also chairman of the board of Cytovance Biologics, the owner of the state's first pharmaceutical manufacturing plant, located in the research park.

Emergent Technologies has launched new funds to assist scientist-entrepreneurs in creating start-up companies and to support technology-based economic development. Nova Venture Services was established to provide private sector capital and consulting services for Oklahoma biotechnology and technology based start-up companies.

InterGenetics, Inc., a genetic cancer risk intervention company, is an innovator in the frontier of genetic medicine. The company has a promising research pipeline of predictive tests for colon, prostate, and ovarian cancer. InterGenetics' core research has future application in predicting heart disease, diabetes, and in making more effective drug therapies and preventative medicine in these fields.

In September, 2008, an advertising campaign was launched to introduce "OU Medicine" as the collective brand name of the OU

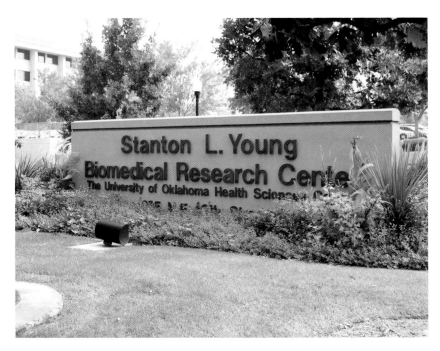

The Stanton L. Young Biomedical Research Center is named for one of the original five Oklahoma City civic leaders who dreamt big. For nearly a half century, Young has supported the idea that became the Oklahoma Health Center. *Courtesy Eric Dabney.*

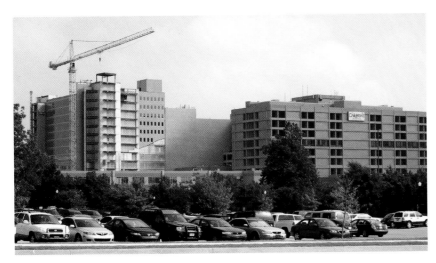

Construction cranes signaled still more construction on the Oklahoma Health Center campus in 2008. *Courtesy Eric Dabney.*

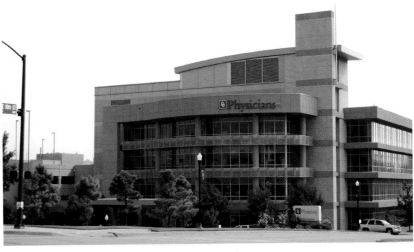

OU Physicians is the state's largest physicians group with more than 450 doctors. The practice encompasses almost every adult and child specialty. *Courtesy Eric Dabney.*

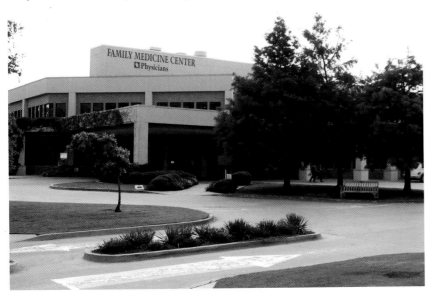

The Family Medicine Center is part of OU Physicians with separate facilities on the Oklahoma Health Center campus. *Courtesy Eric Dabney.*

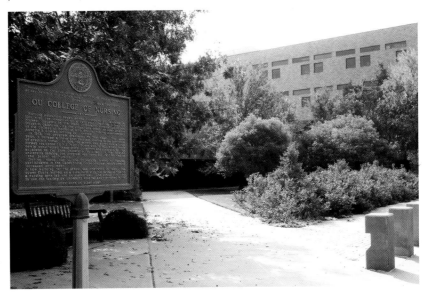

The OU College of Nursing has a long and distinguished record as providing Oklahomans with quality nurse practitioners. Nursing education began at OU in 1911. A bachelor's degree in nursing was authorized beginning in 1951. *Courtesy Eric Dabney.*

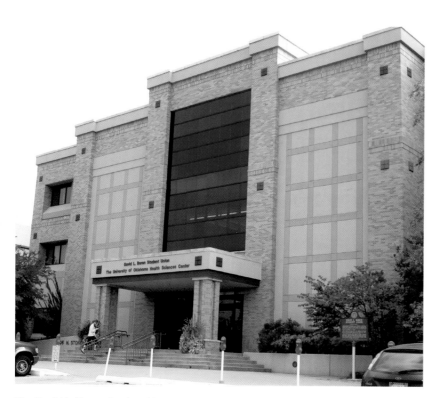

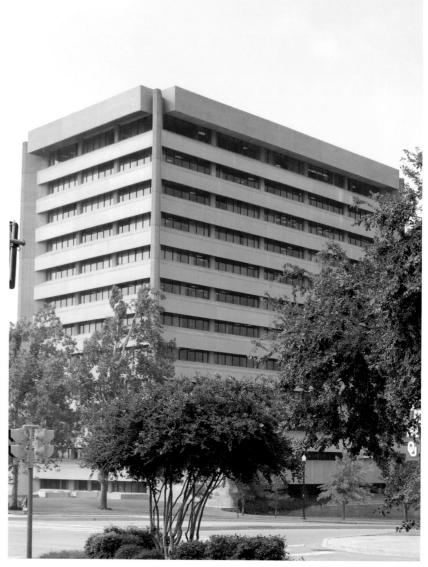

The David L. Boren Student Union is a central gathering point for faculty and students in the professional schools at the OUHSC. *Courtesy Eric Dabney.*

The Oklahoma State Department of Health is responsible for protecting and promoting the health of citizens of Oklahoma. The Oklahoma State Board of Health governs the state agency that occupies one of the first high-rise buildings constructed on the Oklahoma Health Center campus. *Courtesy Eric Dabney.*

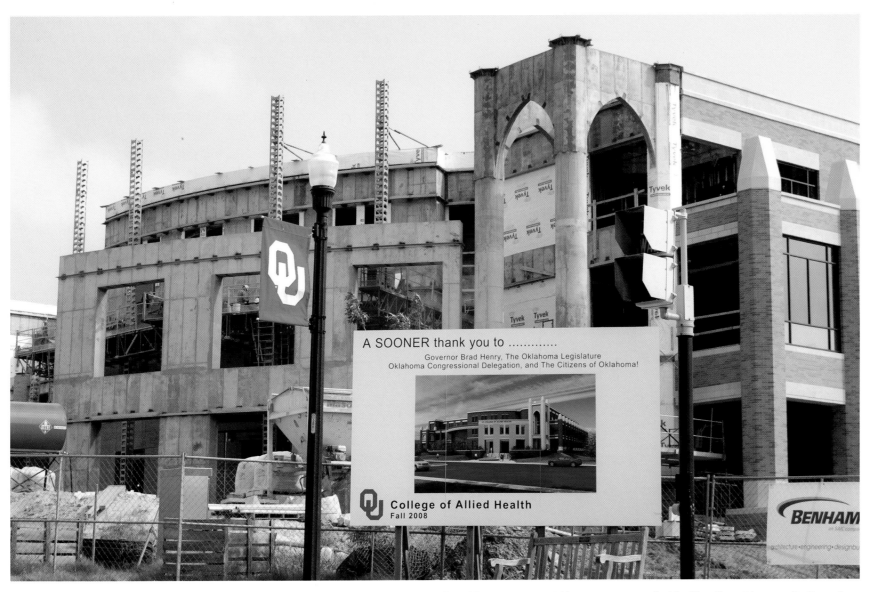

A SOONER thank you to ....

Governor Brad Henry, The Oklahoma Legislature
Oklahoma Congressional Delegation, and The Citizens of Oklahoma!

College of Allied Health
Fall 2008

The OU College of Allied Health Building was one of the latest construction projects on the OUHSC campus in 2008. The 115,000-square-foot facility will provide space for the college to continue to train health professionals and support students who are spread out across the nation and in many foreign countries. *Courtesy Eric Dabney.*

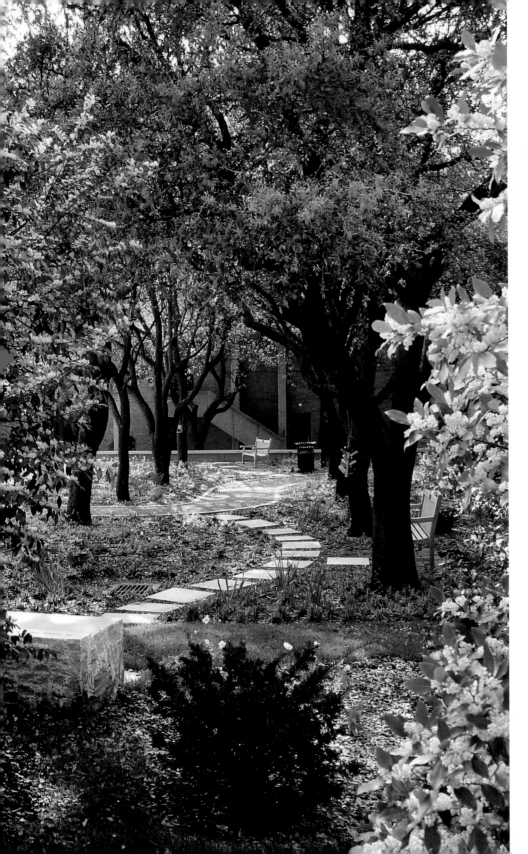

College of Medicine, OU Physicians, and the OU Medical Center, including Children's Hospital, and the University Hospitals Trust. The new brand was intended to eliminate public confusion about how the similarly-named entities on the OHC campus work together. "Another goal," said OU College of Medicine Dean M. Dewayne Andrews, "is to increase visibility and awareness of the quality of care patients can expect from OU Medicine."

A quarter century after it was born, the Oklahoma Health Center concept has become reality. It is a bustling center of ideas, education, medical care, far-reaching research, commercialization, and economic development.

Dr. Joseph Ferretti steered the OUHSC through one of its most expansive periods of growth and achievement, which included new student, research, and clinical buildings, establishment of innovative research programs and record philanthropic support. Amazing progress has been made in the last 20 years as the overall budget increased to more than $600 million annually. Even more impressive is that the OUHSC faculty increased external research seven-fold and NIH research increased 10-fold. At the same time, the substantial progress has been made with only a doubling of state government appropriations. Even though OUHSC is not as large as similar centers in Dallas or Houston, its academic programs are far more comprehensive.

OUHSC is unique among academic health centers for several reasons. The location is spacious and allows for continued expansion of health related activities. Many of the nation's academic medical centers are land-locked in terms of available space for future growth. OHC has had the luxury of available space to attract health and research-related organizations.

The OU College of Medicine and related teaching hospitals are

Fountains and many open air and walking spaces are part of the beautification project at the Oklahoma Health Center. *Courtesy Childrens Medical Research Institute.*

Oklahoma's Veterans Affairs Medical Center

The Veterans Affairs Medical Center (VAMC) in Oklahoma City is a teaching hospital, which allows us to provide a full range of patient care services with state of the art technology. Comprehensive health care is provided through primary care, tertiary care, and long-term care in areas of medicine, surgery, psychiatry, rehabilitation, oncology, dentistry, and geriatrics and extended care, just to name a few. Our geriatrics department was started in 1997, while the extended care unit was added on to the department in 2005. It is one of only ten such units in the nation. It is a well established unit that is here to better serve our veterans in transition from hospital to home, improving the continuum of care for the patient. We offer many specialized programs at our facility including Mental Health Intensive Case Management (MHICM), and Reaching out to Educate and Assist Caring Healthy families (REACH). These programs allow us to offer our veterans the best care, which will enhance their ability to be more productive in the community.

Research is another important aspect of the Oklahoma City VAMC that contributes to enhancing our ability to provide current medical techniques and treatments to our veteran patients through areas of research such as Cardiology, Oncology, Neuromimmunology, and currently there are 152 active research projects conducted here in the Medical Center. Along with making sure that we meet customer satisfaction, we make sure that our employees are working in a comfortable environment that allows them to expand their horizons through various opportunities for growth. The Oklahoma City VAMC actively participates in numerous career development programs that are targeted to advance employee satisfaction and succession planning efforts. Such programs offered are: LDI (Leadership Development Institute), GHATP (Graduate Health Administration Training Program), and EISP (Employee Incentive Scholarship Program).

As one can see, The Oklahoma City VAMC is a hospital with purpose and we provide a magnitude of services to our patient veteran population through providing continuity of care. Quality of care is what we constantly strive to offer our patients, along with commitment and access at a clinical and administrative level. We hope to continue impacting the health community as well as meet a standard of excellence all throughout the Veterans Affairs system, while remaining a driving force here in the Oklahoma City Medical Center community.

David Wood, Director
Veterans Affairs Medical Center, Oklahoma City

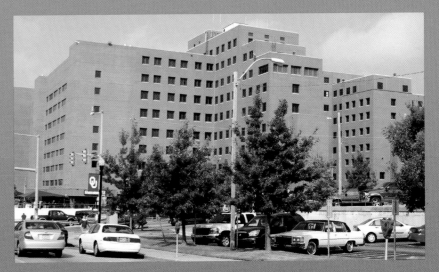

The Oklahoma City Veterans Affairs Medical Center on the Oklahoma Health Center campus serves 48 Oklahoma counties and two counties in north Texas with a veteran population of more than 250,000. The Oklahoma City facility operates a 172-bed teaching hospital, providing a full range of patient care services. *Courtesy Eric Dabney.*

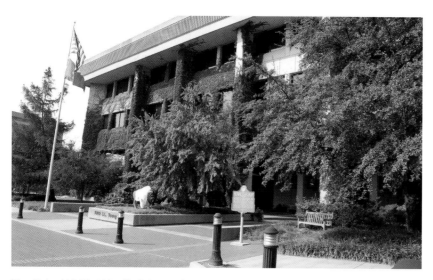

The Robert M. Bird Health Sciences Library is a central building in the OU Health Sciences Center complex. *Courtesy Eric Dabney.*

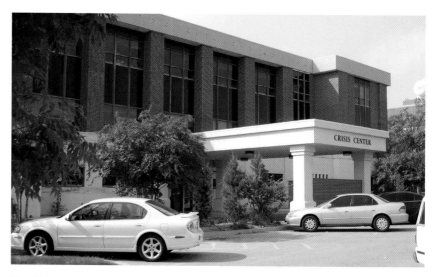

The Oklahoma Department of Mental Health & Substance Abuse operates the Oklahoma County Crisis Intervention Center, one of many programs designed for individuals experiencing problems related to mental illness, substance abuse, domestic violence, and sexual assault. Each year, the agency provides services to nearly 100,000 clients. *Courtesy Eric Dabney.*

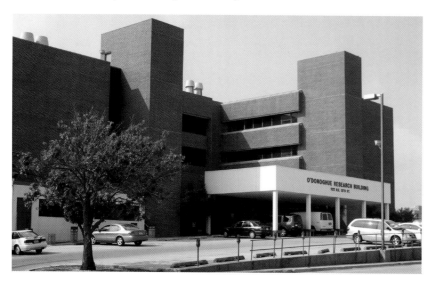

The O'Donoghue Research Building was originally the O'Donoghue Rehabilitation Center, named for Dr. Donald O'Donoghue, one of the original leaders who helped make the Oklahoma Health Center a reality. *Courtesy Eric Dabney.*

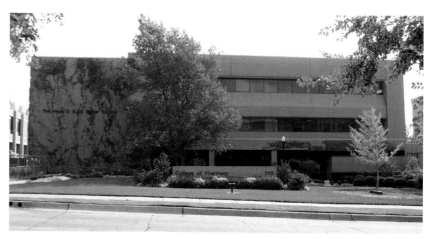

The OU College of Pharmacy is housed in the Henry D. and Ida Mosier Building. The college's faculty members are recognized nationally and internationally for their contributions to teaching, research, and service. *Courtesy Eric Dabney.*

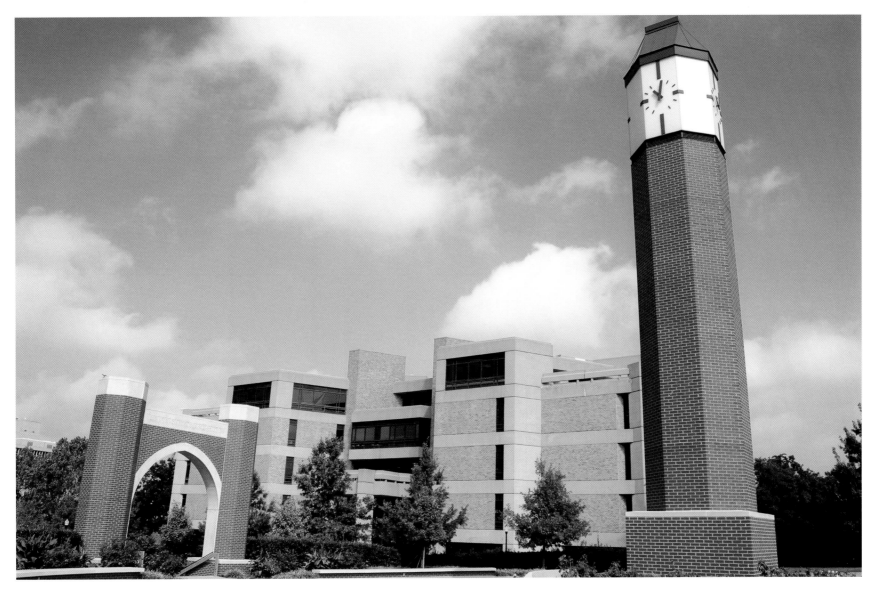

The OU College of Dentistry graduated its first class in 1976. The college currently accepts 58 dental students into each class of the DDS four-year program and dental hygiene students at Oklahoma City and three distance locations. A $9.8 million federal grant in 2003 strengthened the research infrastructure of the college, including the establishment of state-of-the-art laboratory facilities. In the foreground is the Thelma Gaylord Memorial Clock Tower. *Courtesy Eric Dabney.*

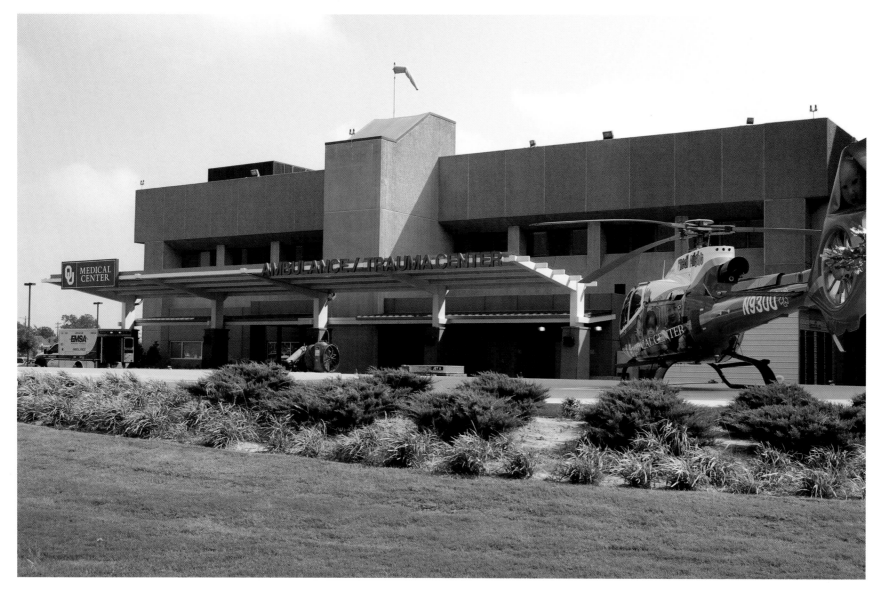

A medically-equipped Medi Flight helicopter delivers an injured Oklahoman to the trauma center at the OU Medical Center. *Courtesy Eric Dabney.*

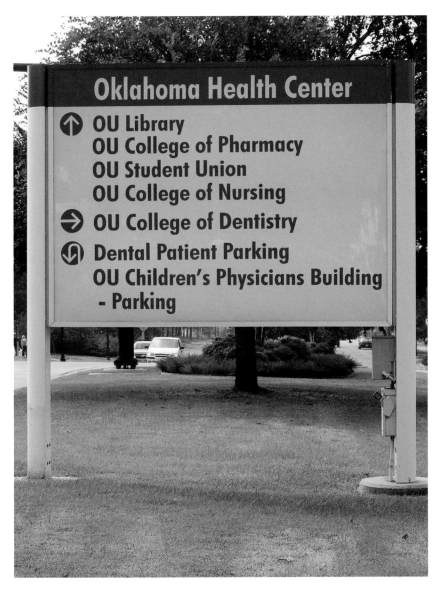

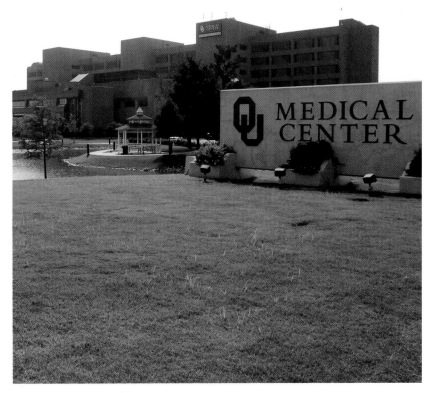

A series of signs on the Oklahoma Health Center campus direct visitors to their intended destinations. *Courtesy Eric Dabney.*

The OU Medical Center is Oklahoma City's largest and most diverse hospital, featuring a winning team of world-class academic and private physicians, nurses, and health care specialists. The names of the former University, Children's, and Presbyterian hospitals were changed to OU Medical Center in 2001. *Courtesy Eric Dabney.*

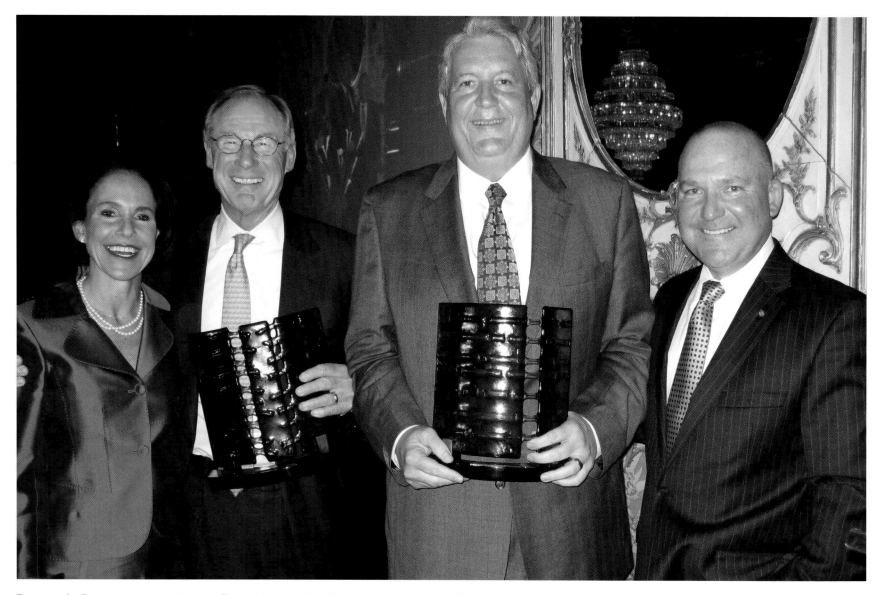

Treasures for Tomorrow event co-chairmen, Susan Edwards, left, and Mark Funke, right, congratulate two of the 2008 honorees, Burns Hargis, second from left, and Michael Turpen. *Courtesy Oklahoma Health Center Foundation.*

a magnet to attract more health organizations to the OHC campus. Availability of common resources and the existence of numerous health professionals, libraries, facilities, and state organizations add to the uniqueness of the campus. Few academic health centers have a research park and state health department, mental health department, medical examiner's office, and other agencies surrounding the teaching hospitals and the Veterans Affairs Medical Center.

Dr. Joseph Ferretti said, "We have 30 organizations working together in critical mass, feeding off of each other. Complimenting and joining these different health and research organizations are kindred groups, such as the Oklahoma Medical Research Foundation, the Presbyterian Health Foundation Research Park, the Oklahoma School for Science and Mathematics—all who like to be near an academic medical complex."

When the Oklahoma Health Center idea was born, the shortage of qualified medical workers was a significant reason civic leaders and elected officials got behind the project. A shortage of health care workers continues to be a major motivator for continued growth. By 2012, Oklahoma is expected to have a shortage of more than 3,000 nurses, 600 lab technicians, 400 physical therapists, 300 surgical technologists, and 200 occupational therapists. Health care industry workers made up 14 percent of the state labor force.

A physician shortage is also expected in the next decade. A recent report showed the country will experience a 20 percent shortfall of physicians, 200,000 fewer than needed. Primary care specialists will be most in demand. The OU professional schools are aware of the predictions and are increasing enrollment to help meet the need. Statistically, doctors tend to remain in the area where they train, so increasing the number of physicians-in-training in

Oklahoma is essential to increasing the workforce.

Improving the health of all Oklahomans is a primary goal of expanding the Oklahoma Health Center. The rapid expansion of the diabetes and cancer research and treatment programs at OUHSC, coupled with exponential growth in research investment are fundamental to the health of state citizens. With increased medical services available, no longer is it necessary for Oklahomans to go outside the state's borders for the latest treatment.

An example of cutting-edge technology used to help Oklahomans is proton therapy, a cancer treatment using proton beams to precisely target tumors. Research shows proton beams cause less damage to tissue surrounding a cancerous tumor. Proton therapy will be a major emphasis in cancer treatment at the OU Cancer Institute.

OU Physicians employs more than 450 doctors and offers every conceivable subspecialty. Brian Maddy, CEO of OU Physicians, said, "We treat the tiniest high-risk babies to the sickest of our elderly citizens. We also care for every part of a person's body. We now have an excellent group of physicians that literally nurture Oklahomans from cradle to grave."

Maddy explained the benefits of the combined teaching and patient care missions for OU Physicians:

Our patients get the best of both worlds. They are treated by a doctor who is teaching the next generation of physicians. The patient benefits from the richness of the teacher's wisdom and experience and the excitement of the student who is learning and testing the newest treatments and ideas. It is a special moment to observe the steady hand of the experienced physician guiding the students, listening to their questions, and helping them think through what is best for the patient.

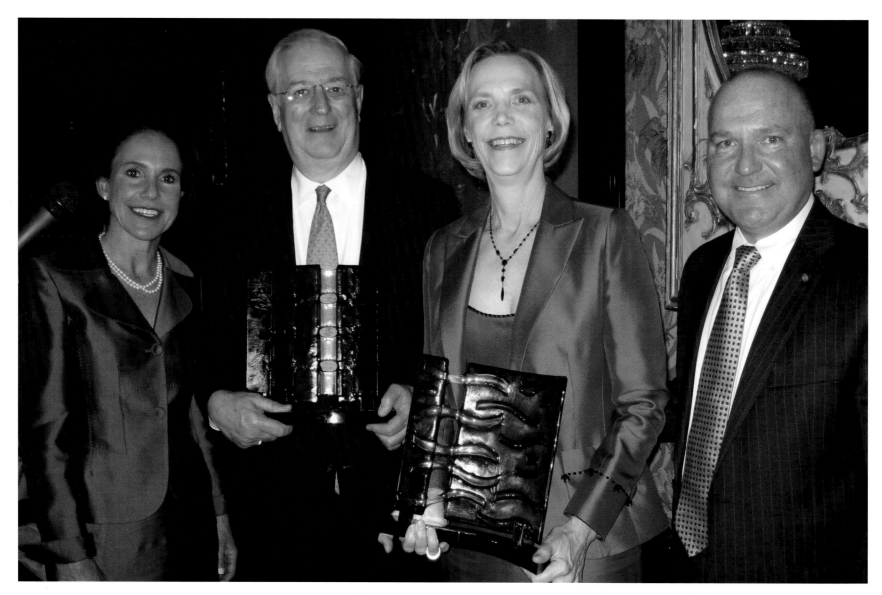

OUHSC Provost Dr. Joseph Ferretti and his wife, Martha "Marti" Ferretti, were among the 2008 recipients of the Treasures for tomorrow award. Shown with the Ferrettis are event co-chair Susan Edwards, left, and Mark Funke, right. *Courtesy Oklahoma Health Center Foundation.*

There are examples of a "triple threat" on the OUHSC campus—physicians who see patients as a clinician, teach medical students and residents, and conduct research. Much of the research is transitional, in which the newest drugs and technology are evaluated for safety and efficiency.

The comprehensive approach to medical research, education, and patient treatment on the OHC campus enhances the fundamental commitment to excellent health care. Dr. Ferretti said: When patients visit OUHSC, they may experience the academic health center difference in only very subtle ways. However, they can rest assured that our foundation is built upon uniting physicians of many different specialties to provide a comprehensive approach to health care. Discoveries made on our campus by renowned researchers make their way into everyday care sooner and are readily available to patients. That makes a tremendous difference in how we prevent illness, identify the causes of health conditions, and treat challenging diseases.

In all parts of the OHC campus, excellence and action combine to continually improve and expand services to Oklahomans. Some programs are large, such as the Oklahoma Medical Research Foundation, Dean A. McGee Eye Institute, or the Oklahoma Blood Institute which was the first blood center in the nation to provide cholesterol and HIV Antigen testing on donated blood. OBI is the seventh largest non-profit regional blood center in the United States, collecting more than 250,000 donated blood units each year.

Other OHC programs are small. The Oklahoma Health Center Clinical Pastoral Education Institute, primarily funded by the Presbyterian Health Foundation , is dedicated to training professionals who can integrate religion and health for patients in hospitals and other health care facilities. Some of the start-up companies in the PHF Research Park have only a skeleton staff—for now. As Hershel Lamirand said, "The ideas being generated from the OHC campus will surely lead to a brighter tomorrow for Oklahoma's economy, but more importantly, for Oklahoma's people."

Stanton L. Young has been a constant observer of and strong advocate for the growth and development of the Oklahoma Health Center. He was at the initial meetings nearly a half century ago when leaders dared to look beyond budget constraints and naysayers and dream of a vibrant, world-class medical and research center that would accomplish all the stated goals—and more. Young, never one to rest on his past accomplishments, said, "We have only scratched the surface of our potential. There is no limit to the good things coming from this plot of ground that was renewed beyond our wildest dreams."

Oklahoma Health Center Foundation

The Future of Oklahoma Health Center

It is difficult to restrain my enthusiasm for the future of the Oklahoma Health Center. One only has to review the history of the institutions that make up the OHC to realize what incredible potential lies in the decades ahead. Significant progress has been made in health care, education, technology, and research. The economy of the state has been given an unprecedented boost. However, the OHC is just getting started!

In the next few years OHC's physicians, teachers, researchers, and entrepreneurs will literally change life in the world. Media will report significant breakthroughs in diagnosing and limiting the effect of debilitating diseases upon the world's population. As methods of treatment and innovate drugs are developed on the OHC campus, quality of life will advance—a most worthy goal.

When another generation looks back at the Oklahoma Health Center's progress in the first decades of the twenty-first century, I am confident they will wholeheartedly agree that OHC institutions had a huge effect on growing the Oklahoma economy and made a positive contribution to the health of welfare of all Oklahomans and citizens of the world. OHC is making a difference—one life at a time.

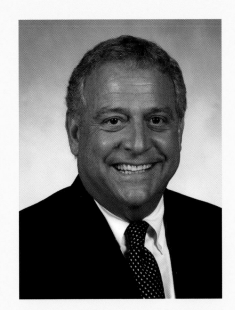

Hershel Lamirand is president of the Oklahoma Health Center Foundation.

W. Hershel Lamirand, III
President, Oklahoma Health Center Foundation

Board of Directors, 2009

Ann Ackerman, Ph.D.
Chief Executive Officer
Leadership Oklahoma

M. Dewayne Andrews, M.D.
Vice President for Health Affairs
& Executive Dean, College of Medicine
University of Oklahoma Health Sciences Center

William M. Bell
Vice Chairman
BancFirst

Lance Benham
Principal
The Benham Companies

Clayton I. Bennett
President
Dorchester Capital

David Bialis
President,
Cox Communications–Oklahoma

David L. Boren
President
The University of Oklahoma

John R. Bozalis, M.D.
Oklahoma Allergy & Asthma Clinic

Ronald E. Bradshaw
President
Ron E. Bradshaw and Co.

JoeVan Bullard
Executive Director
Oklahoma City Urban Renewal Authority

James D. Couch
City Manager
City of Oklahoma City

Douglas R. Cummings
Chairman
Cummings Oil Co.

Bruce W. Day
Partner
Day, Edwards, Propester & Christenson, P.C.

Carl E. Edwards
Managing Partner
Price Edwards & Co.

James H. Everest
General Partner
Everest Brothers

Mike Fogarty
Chief Executive Officer
Oklahoma Health Care Authority

Mark W. Funke
President
Bank of Oklahoma

Bryan Gonterman
President
AT&T Oklahoma

David R. Harlow
President
BancFirst

Danny P. Harris
Sr. Vice President and Chief Operating Officer
OGE Energy Corporation

Howard H. Hendrick
Director
Oklahoma Department of Human Services

G.P. Johnson Hightower
Senior Vice President & Senior Trust Officer
Stillwater National Bank & Trust Co.

Henry J. Hood
Senior Vice President
Land and Legal and General Counsel
Chesapeake Energy Corporation

Bob Howard
President
Mercedes-Benz of Oklahoma City

Sue Ann Hyde

Jane Jenkins
President
Downtown Oklahoma City

Michael E. Joseph
Lawyer
McAfee & Taft

Ronald "Skip" Kelly
Oklahoma City Council, Ward 7
City of Oklahoma City

Lou C. Kerr
President and Vice Chair
The Kerr Foundation, Inc.

William C. Liedtke III
Vice President and General Counsel
Windsor Energy Resources, Inc.

Dave Lopez
President
American Fidelity Foundation

Mary Mélon
Publisher
Journal Record

Garrett F. "Bud" Miles
Principal
Miles Associates Incorporated

Roger Mitchell
President
Oklahoma Natural Gas

Bradley Z. Naifeh
Owner
Central Liquor Company

Bond Payne
Chairman
Heritage Trust Company

Cathy Perri
Senior Coordinator, Oklahoma GEAR UP
Oklahoma State Regents for Higher Education

Kevin Perry
Vice President
Perry Publishing & Broadcasting

James A. Pickel
Vice President
Smith & Pickel Construction

William N. Pirtle

David E. Rainbolt
President and Chief Executive Officer
BancFirst Corporation

Charlotte Richels

Patrick T. Rooney
Chairman and CEO
First National Bank of Oklahoma

Robert J. Ross
President and CEO
Inasmuch Foundation and
Excellence in Journalism Foundation

Michael S. Samis
President
Samis Investments, LLC

Natalie Shirley
Director
Oklahoma Department of Commerce

David Thompson
President & Publisher
OPUBCO Communications Group

Gena Timberman
Executive Director
Native American Cultural & Educational
Authority/American Indian Cultural Center &
Museum

Carol Troy
Senior Vice President
Saxum Public Relations

Ty Tyler
President
Tyler Media

Roy H. Williams
President
Greater Okla City Chamber

G. Rainey Williams Jr.
President
Marco Capital Group

Stanton L. Young
President
The Young Companies

Chief Executive Officers

Michael Anderson, Ph.D.
President
Presbyterian Health Foundation

John Armitage, M.D.
President and Chief Executive Officer
Sylvan N. Goldman Center/
Oklahoma Blood Institute

John M. Bell, M.D.
President
Oklahoma City Clinic

Rev. Ken Blank
Executive Director
Oklahoma Health Center Clinical Pastoral
Education Institute, Inc.

William M. Canfield, M.D., Ph.D.
President
Genzyme
and
Nova Ventures Services, LLC

Mike Carolina
Executive Director
Oklahoma Center for the Advancement of
Science & Technology (OCAST)

Eric Duval, D.O.
Interim Chief Medical Examiner
Office of the Chief Medical Examiner

Cole Eslyn FACHE
President and CEO
OU MEDICAL CENTER

Joseph J. Ferretti, Ph.D.
Senior Vice President and Provost
OU Health Sciences Center

Dean Gandy
Executive Director
University Hospitals Authority and Trust

Herb Gilkey
Director
Ronald McDonald House

Darren Head
President & CEO
Cytovance Biologics

Vincent Hernandez
Chief Executive Officer
American Red Cross of Central Oklahoma

John Hoopingarner
Chief Operating Officer
Emergent Technologies, Inc.

Tom Kupiec, Ph.D.
President and CEO
ARL Bio Pharma, Inc.

W. Hershel Lamirand III
President
Oklahoma Health Center Foundation

Brian L. Maddy
Chief Executive Officer
OU Physicians

Edna M. Manning, Ed.D.
President
Oklahoma School of Science
and Mathematics

Kathlene C. McCracken
Executive Director
Children's Medical Research Institute

Rocky McElvany
Interim Commissioner of Health
Oklahoma State Department of Health

David W. Parke II, M.D.
President and Chief Executive Officer
Dean McGee Eye Institute

Paula Porter
President
Easter Seals Oklahoma

Stephen M. Prescott, M.D.
President
Oklahoma Medical Research
Foundation

Joseph A. Schraad MHA
Chief Operating Officer
Oklahoma Allergy & Asthma Clinic

Denise Semands Suttles
President and CEO
GlobalHealth, Inc.

Tom Walker
President and Chief Executive Officer
i2E, Inc.

Terri White
ODMHSAS Commissioner
Oklahoma Department of Mental Health & Substance Abuse Services

David P. Wood, FACHE
Director
Department of Veterans Affairs Medical Center

Staff

W. Hershel Lamirand III
President

Terry Taylor
Planning and Operations Director

Mary Kay Audd
Staff Assistant